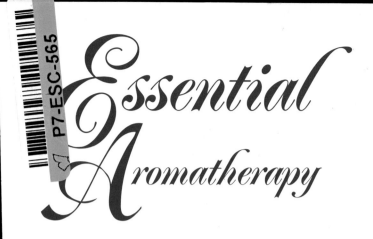

Essential Aromatherapy

A POCKET GUIDE

to

ESSENTIAL OILS

&

AROMATHERAPY

Susan E. Worwood

NEW WORLD LIBRARY
SAN RAFAEL, CALIFORNIA

Published by New World Library
58 Paul Drive
San Rafael, California, 94903
Copyright © 1995 by Affirmative Books Ltd.

Cover painting: Chantal Saperstein
Illustrator: Edwina Hannam
Design & typography: Stephanie Eichleay
Editorial & production: Becky Benenate

Library of Congress Cataloging-in-Publication Data

Worwood, Susan E., 1955–
Essential aromatherapy : a pocket guide to essential oils
and aromatherapy / by Susan E. Worwood
p.   cm.   Includes biographical references and index.
ISBN 1-880032-66-X (pbk. : alk. paper)
1. Aromatherapy — Handbooks, manuals, etc.   2. Essences
and essential oils — Handbooks, manuals, etc.   I. Title.
RM666.A68W65   1995   95-4563
615'.321 — dc20   CIP

First printing September, 1995
Printed in the U.S.A.
10 9 8 7 6 5 4 3 2 1

Dedication

This book is dedicated to my son, Michael,
for all the love and joy he brings me.

Acknowledgments

J would like to thank the following people for their help and encouragement: my sister, Valerie Ann Worwood, who has shared her research and knowledge of aromatherapy and essential oils; Clive Bendon for the use of his library and sharing his expertise in essential oil analysis; Julia Stonehouse for her support with Essentially Yours Ltd; and my mother, Vera, for her constant love and support in all I attempt. Finally, I thank all the aromatherapists whose work and persistence over many years has made aromatherapy a household word, known the world over, and who continue to bring help to so many people in so many ways.

Contents

Glossary of the Therapeutic Uses of
Essential Oils
The Chemistry of Essential Oils
Individual Essential Oil Profiles
Purchasing guide, Color , Viscosity, Aroma,
Countries of origin, Description (of plant),
Part used, Extraction method, Yield, Most
valuable uses, Therapeutic properties, Main
chemical components, Blends well with,
Interesting facts, Contraindications
Individual Essential Oils
*Basil, Bay, Benzoin, Bergamot, Black Pepper,
Cardamom, Carnation, Cedarwood,
Chamomile German, Chamomile Roman,
Cinnamon, Clary Sage, Clove, Coriander,
Cypress, Eucalyptus Citriodora, Eucalyptus
Globulus, Eucalyptus Radiata, Fennel,
Frankincense, Geranium, Ginger, Grapefruit,
Helichrysum, Hyacinth, Jasmine, Juniper,
Lavender, Lemon, Lemongrass, Linden
Blossom, Litsea Cubeba, Mandarin, Manuka,
Marjoram, Melissa, Myrrh, Neroli, Orange,
Oregano, Ormenis Flower, Palmarosa,
Patchouli, Peppermint, Petitgrain, Pine,
Ravensara, Rose Maroc, Rose Otto, Rosemary,
Sandalwood, Spikenard, Tagetes, Tea Tree,
Thyme, Vetiver, Ylang Ylang, Yuzu*

Introduction

$\mathscr{E}$ssential oils are part of American history. When doctor and pharmacist John Pemberton invented Coca-Cola in May 1886, he flavored his new "nerve tonic" with the essential oils of orange, lemon, nutmeg, cinnamon, coriander, and neroli. The "flavorings" portion of the drink's formula is known as "7X," raising the question, what was the seventh ingredient? It has been suggested that it was the extract of vanilla, known to be included in the complete formula, or that it was lime oil. It has even been suggested that lavender oil was a component of the drink.[1] Since the exact formula of Coca-Cola is a trade secret, we cannot say exactly which essential oils are contained in it today. What we do know is that without essential oils, the food and beverage industries of the entire world would be at a very serious loss. You only have to look at the list of ingredients on the products in any supermarket to see that essential oils are universal. As peppermint and spearmint, essential oils are even in that

---

[1]Mark Pendergrast, *For God, Country and Coca-Cola*, London: Weidenfeld and Nicolson, 1993, pp. 422-424; William Poundstone, *Big Secrets*, New York: Quill, 1983, pp. 42-43.

other quintessentially American product, chewing gum.

Essential oils are also used extensively in the perfume, cosmetics, and toiletries industries. These days, especially, customers demand natural purity, and as a result many advertisers are keen to stress the fact that their products include essential oils. This aspect of their use is extremely old, and beauties from the earliest times employed the considerable benefits of plant essences to enhance their chances in love. Cleopatra, Queen of Egypt, even went so far as to soak the sails of her royal barge in rose essence so that the aroma would drift on the wind and announce her imminent arrival to Anthony, waiting farther down the River Nile to greet her.

Royal women have always appreciated the benefits of essential oils and been in the position to ensure their supply of them. Cleopatra kept vast gardens expressly for that purpose. In the sixteenth century, Elizabeth I, Queen of England, used copious amounts of lavender oil, as did Queen Victoria in the nineteenth century — the former no doubt to keep bugs of all descriptions at bay, while the latter needed all the help she could get to see her through her record-breaking sixty-four year reign. Both appreciated the fact that lavender grows well in the Norfolk fields. Today, British royals extol the virtues of natural medicines, with various members using them regularly. Princess Diana, for example, is often reported in the press as having been on her way to, or coming from, an aromatherapy treatment. No doubt, with all the stress in her life, essential oils are much appreciated!

As medicines, essential oils appeared in the first pharmacopoeias. Although their use has been replaced over recent years by chemical copies or replacements, some still appear in their original form, while others have been given more scientific-sounding names. Medical scientists, perhaps more than anyone else, appreciate the benefits of nature's rich and varied bounty. Indeed, as the rain forests and other natural habitats continue to be depleted, laboratories all over the world are rushing to send groups of researchers into less-developed regions of the world to gather medicinal information that is in danger of being lost, in search of cures for the future.

Essential oils, then, are nothing new. They are not a passing fad, but an ancient and enduring harvest of nature's richness. In previous times, there was nothing to prove that essential oils worked, except people's actual day-to-day experience. Today, laboratories put essential oils through batteries of tests and the results are published in academic journals. This process is not at all complete. Experience, however, defines reality, and the reality is essential oils, used correctly, work. Science will, with time, continue to prove this point.

Let us never forget that nature is resplendent with life-giving gifts. Trees stand magnificently on the horizon, silently pumping gasses into the atmosphere, creating the pure air we need to breathe. Plants of all shapes and sizes offer us their fruits, their produce, upon which our sustenance depends. Other plants support animals, which in turn become vital food sources for other animals. Without plants we would neither eat nor breathe; we depend totally upon them.

We also spice our food with herbs, sometimes unaware how much good they do us. And we perfume our world with delightful scents provided by spices and flowers, grasses, leaves, barks, and even resin oozing from the bark; while the sight of colorful flowers stuns us with their beauty. How flat life would be without these special gifts.

Throughout history, people have turned to nature to provide help during illness. In many parts of the world today, from Africa to Europe, bunches of varied herbs are sold in markets, as they have been for untold centuries. Medicinal herbal teas are probably known in all countries, with some cultures employing them more than others. In countries where there are no doctors nearby, children are taught when they cut themselves to pick the leaves of a particular plant to cover the wound and prevent infection. Other children follow their mothers as they gather roots, barks, grasses, flowers, leaves, and other plant parts that will be used to cure the sick. Some of these materials have traditionally been made into essential oils which, in almost every country of the world, have formed an integral part of the materia medica of ordinary people.

We are a fortunate generation because we can take advantage not only of nature itself — and future generations may not have that chance — but we can also assemble information concerning the efficacy of plants and their essential oils and broadly communicate that information. This can even be done instantaneously and sent to the other side of the world via computer networks. As we enter the third millennium, we can draw upon science to help us better understand the source of all plants, and ask it to guide us so we may take full advantage of the vital gifts that plants generously offer us.

Chapter 1

ESSENTIAL OILS, NATURE'S ESSENCE

Essential oils are concentrated plant essences. Although they are called "oils," this is something of a misnomer because most essential oils are not in fact oily, unlike vegetable oils which have been expressed from seeds or plant nuts (such as sesame, sunflower, peach kernel, and sweet almond). A few essential oils are rather viscous and others are fairly solid. Most, however, are watery, with lavender, lemon, and eucalyptus being classic examples. The color of essential oils varies, tending to be clear or yellow, although carrot is orange, spikenard is green, and chamomile german a beautiful deep blue. Of course, essential oils are characterized most of all by their individual aromas — hence the term "aromatherapy."

Essential oils are derived from relatively few plants and, depending on the variety, only from particular parts of that plant. These include the leaves, roots, buds, twigs, rhizomes, heartwood, bark, resin, flower petals, seeds, or fruit. In some cases the whole of the plant that grows above ground is used, as in peppermint, for example. There is a huge variation in the price of different essential oils reflecting, above all, the volume of material available, but also transportation costs and growing conditions in any given year. It takes vast quantities of hand-picked, tiny jasmine petals to produce a few drops of jasmine oil while tea tree oil can be produced much more cheaply using mechanical methods to harvest the leaves of that plant. All essential oil-producing plants are different in their yield, as well. Clary sage, for example, yields 0.3-1% essential oil, while clove yields 10-15%. From the same volume of material, then, clove produces up to forty-five times more essential oil than clary sage.

Throughout the world, there are approximately 3,000 essential oils, most of which are used only in the local regions in which they are found. About 300 are in more general use, and are traded world-wide. It is helpful to know where a particular oil comes from because, for example, geranium oils grown in Egypt, China, or Reunion each have their unique characteristics. Also, the same species of plant will produce an oil with different properties depending on whether it was grown in dry or damp earth, for example, or at high or low altitude, or in a hot or cold climate.

Some essential oils contain hundreds of biochemical components, while others have only a few. And some components are present in quite large proportions while many others are present only in traces. The analysis of essential oils is still at the stage where we cannot yet say exactly how many components are in any particular essential oil, because all small traces have not been identified. Indeed, they cannot be registered because the means of analysis are not yet available. Each essential oil has a unique fingerprint, and we cannot fully identify that fingerprint because parts of it are not yet "on file" — the components are simply unknown. As methods of analysis become ever more sophisticated, and as the scientific world's catalog of components enlarges, more and more ingredients will become identifiable.

The therapeutic action of essential oils is usually attributed to the naturally occurring chemicals found within them. Within the essential oil of yuzu (*Citrus junos*), for example, there are known to be 124 compounds, comprised of 44 alcohols, 26 hydrocarbons, 12 esters, 9 ketones, 14 aldehydes, 3 phenols and 16 miscellaneous others.[2] Other terms in the vocabulary of essential oil analysis include terpenes, coumarines, acids, ethers, and sesquiterpenes. The way these various natural chemicals interact with each other gives an essential oil its unique qualities and, some would say,

---

[2]Volatile Components of Yuzu (Citrus Junos), Ichiro Watanabe et al., *Flavours and Fragrance*

explains its therapeutic properties. Alcohols can be shown to be antibacterial, for example, and coumarins sedative. (See Chapter 8).

Various methods are used to establish the compounds in essential oils. The best form of analysis involves using several procedures in conjunction to establish the chemical components and their purity. Capillary gas liquid chromatography establishes the chemical components, while optical rotation establishes whether the essential oil has the correct optical activity — measured in terms of percentages of bend to right or left, or "dextrorotatory" and "laevorotatory" respectively. Also, the specific gravity of the material is measured to establish that it has the correct weight, and the refractive index establishes whether the material reflects the correct angle of sodium light. Together, these tests can establish the purity of the essential oil.

Extraction

The art of extracting the essential oil from plant materials is as old as history itself. It is difficult for us now to imagine the importance of essential oils to our ancestors who relied upon them heavily for medicinal and ritual purposes, as well as for perfume. Indeed, much of the trade in ancient times involved essential oils, which were often prepared then as "unguents" (soothing or healing salves). According to archaeologist Jacquetta Hawkes, "Everybody used them" in ancient Egypt, not just the Pharaohs and other dignitaries. In the lists of products important enough to be included in ancient Egyptian records, over thirty different forms of unguents are mentioned.[3] One method of extraction employed by the Egyptians involved squeezing the plant material, such as lily flowers, in fine linen, which was held secure on a frame at one end and twisted at the other end by a group of people. They also steeped aromatic plant materials in oils and fats of various sorts which, when solid, were sometimes formed into balls or cones, and were commonly used as head or hair decorations. These decorations would slowly melt in the heat and drip down the braided hair, both conditioning the hair and perfuming the air — an ancient "time release" air freshener!

Today, by far the majority of essential oils are produced by steam distillation, which involves putting the plant material in a large closed container known as a vat, and forcing steam through it. The heat and pressure releases the tiny droplets of essential oil from the plant, which then rise with the steam out through a spiral tube known as a condenser. The condenser cools the steam, turning it to liquid. Then the oil and water are separated. Throughout the world there are many variations of steam or water distillation, such as open fire stills, but the principle remains the same — to isolate the essential oil molecules from the plant material.

The art of distillation requires accurately judging the correct combination of heat and pressure of the steam, and the length of time the plant material is subjected to it. If the steam is too hot, the essential oil can be burned. If the pressure is too high, the properties of

---

[3]Jacquetta Hawkes, *The First Great Civilizations*, London: Hutchinson, 1973, page 358.

the essential oil can be destroyed, causing the quality of the product to be reduced. Some delicate plant materials need to be exposed to long periods of very gentle steam pressure, while more robust material can be effectively distilled in shorter periods using higher temperatures and pressure.

So-called "rose water" or "lavender water" are by-products of this distillation process — they are the water from which the essential oil has been separated. During the distillation process the water becomes imbued with the aroma of the plant material. This is sold under the French name of "hydrolats."

Enfleurage is a very old method of extracting essential oils, not used much today because it's very labor-intensive and time consuming. There are several versions of enfleurage which involve immersing the flower petals in a fat so that the fat pulls the essential oil from the petal and becomes saturated with it. Then the fat and essential oil are separated. Because people today do not like essential oils to come into contact with animal matter, the fats now used are usually of vegetable origin, such as cocoa butter or coconut.

One method of enfleurage involves wiping fat on both sides of glass plates, then placing flowers on them to create a tier of fat-covered glass, supported by wooden frames or "chassis." It takes quite a bit of time for the oil to be drawn from the petals — about 24 hours in the case of jasmine and two to three days for tuberose. The glass is then taken off the chassis and the petals are removed, to be replaced with fresh flowers. The process is repeated over and over again until the fat is completely saturated. To extract the essential oil from the fat, a solvent is required — usually a natural alcohol — which is completely evaporated, leaving behind only the essential oil. Such essential oils are called "absolutes."

Enflueurage is still used in some places and is excellent for extracting the essential oil "absolute" from delicate flower petals. Because this process is so labor-intensive, "absolutes" produced by enfleurage are usually very expensive.

A variation on enfleurage is *maceration.* This also involves the use of a liquid fat or oil but in this case the fat or oil is heated to a temperature of about 60 degrees Fahrenheit. The essential-oil material, which may be flowers but could also be leaves and twigs, is put in a glass container full of the fat or oil, and exposed to heat. This breaks down the plant cells containing the essential oil, which is then released into the fat or oil. The plant material is then sifted out and more fresh plant material is added. The process is repeated, sometimes for as long as a month, until the base material is completely saturated. Then, as with enfleurage, it is subjected to solvent extraction to separate the fat or oil from the essential oil.

Expression is the method employed to extract essential oils from the oil sacs contained in the rinds of fruit such as orange, lemon, bergamot, mandarin, and tangerine. In times past this was a very labor-intensive process, involving pressing sponges into the rind, which absorbed the essential oil, and were then squeezed out. Today it is done by machines.

Solvent extraction is often used for gums and resins, but also for other plant materials. It involves covering the plant material in a solvent, which may be a petrochemical, and then extracting the essential oil by filtering the plant material and evaporating the solvent. While this method may be perfectly acceptable to the perfume trade, good aromatherapy companies try to avoid buying essential oils produced using petrochemical solvents.

Plant materials are also processed under low temperatures using CO_2 (carbon dioxide) extraction, in which the essential oil can be produced without impairing the odor of the flowers. Essential oils produced in this way are usually expensive.

Chapter 2

How Essential Oils Work

In aromatherapy there are two basic ways in which essential oils have an effect upon the human body: through the nose and through the skin. Aromas are volatile, meaning they disperse in the air, float, and eventually reach the nose. These aromatic molecules float up the nostrils and come into contact with nerves extending from the olfactory bulbs, and ending in two small, sticky patches at the top of the nasal cavity. When the aroma molecule hits receptors in these nerve-rich patches, it sets off a reaction that results in brain activity. This phenomenon has been observed through brain scans and other imaging techniques.

We sometimes use our mouth when we

inhale. In this case the aroma molecules enter the mouth, an excellent absorption medium because it is full of delicate mucus membrane. Aromatic molecules can enter the bloodstream in this way or through the mucus membrane of the nasal cavity. The absorption potential of these two areas of the body is increasingly being explored by doctors and pharmaceutical companies, who now make preparations that are sniffed or taken sublingually — under the tongue. It is difficult to say whether a particular oil is working specifically on the olfactory nerve path system or being absorbed through mucus membrane into the bloodstream. Essential oil molecules also enter the trachea and lungs as we inhale.

Essential oils are also thought to enter the body through the skin because their molecules are extremely tiny. The surest evidence that essential oils get into the body is found in the scientific analysis of the means of excretion — perspiration, feces, urine, breath — after a certain amount of time has passed following the application of essential oils. Some oils seem to be excreted by one method while others seem to be excreted by another. For example, sandalwood can be detected in urine, which may indicate that this oil works on the urinary system, including the bladder; while garlic is exhaled with the out-breath. It is very interesting that one essential oil appears to naturally find one method of getting out of the body, while another oil finds another route. It may well be that all oils are excreted in all the usual manners, but to differing degrees in each.

When using essential oils on the body, whether as a massage oil or in baths, we are still utilizing the nasal/olfactory route, due to the fact that aromatic molecules are volatile and float around in the air as we receive a massage or take the bath. Also, depending on the particular method used, other routes of entry may be involved. Let us look briefly at these methods of entry in detail, and speculate on how the essential oils may work.

The Sense of Smell

Our brain responds to smells very quickly because our life may depend on it. When smoke from another room reaches our nose and our brain responds by say-ing "fire!", we leap up and rush to attend to it. Smells warn us when food is bad or danger is near. The brain also responds to good smells — babies snuggle into their mothers' familiar breasts. Recognizing the smell and knowing safety and food are near, they relax and fall asleep. As children we build up a memory bank of aromas, some of which have good connotations, and some bad. If home life was happy and mother baked pies with cinnamon, the aroma of that spice will, in later life, evoke memories of times spent happily around the kitchen table. If a child was looked after by indifferent parents who wore lemon-scented perfumes, that aroma will, in later life, bring back uncomfortable, perhaps vague, memories and the aroma will be avoid-ed. In this way, each of us develops an individual aroma history, which continues to develop with time.

Over and above our individual histories with

aromas, there are certain *types* of aroma. Classifying these types has proved difficult because the human nose can distinguish between 10,000 different smells, and that indicates there's a very complex mystery for science to unravel. As of this writing, the exact mechanism for olfaction has not yet been discovered. Some olfactory nerve receptors have been identified, but the process has not been observed experimentally. We know proteins are involved and that, basically, the aroma molecules set off reactions in the brain. The connection is as follows: the aroma molecule hits receptors on small hair-like cilia which extend downwards from the two olfactory bulbs, spoon-like protrusions which are part of the brain. These olfactory bulbs give us our most direct and quickest access to the brain — through aroma.

The part of the brain that most directly responds to olfactory stimulus is the limbic system, which corresponds to our feelings, memories, stored learned responses, and emotions. The limbic system is the most ancient part of the brain, the central core over which the cerebral cortex lies. When aromatic messages reach the limbic system they are processed instantly and instinctively. This is why aromas are so powerful. They can make us behave in particular ways, without us even knowing what we are doing. In an experiment by Dr. Alan Hirsch of the Smell & Taste Treatment and Research Foundation, Chicago, sweet aromas were put around particular gambling machines in Las Vegas and people responded by putting more money in those machines. The management liked the experiment, you can be sure.[4]

Today, olfactory manipulation is far more than an experiment, it is a part of daily life. In banks in Japan, keyboard operators working in large buildings are perked up in the afternoon by the aroma of lemon being diffused into the working environment. The new school of Japanese architecture, which designs for the perfect working environment, recommends commercial diffusion systems capable of diffusing a variety of different aromas into different areas of the workplace, throughout the day. To calm worried relatives, at least one hospital in America has essential oils diffused in the waiting areas. An increasing number of hotels and retail outlets pump both natural and synthetic aromas into the atmosphere to make people relaxed, so they feel like staying longer (or coming back another time) while spending more money. Marketers in the olfaction field are fond of saying that aroma-psychology is the new frontier in the business. (See *The Fragrant Mind* by Valerie Ann Worwood).

Because the olfaction system is linked directly to the brain, essential oils will obviously have an effect upon it, but olfaction also involves other body systems as well. For untold centuries people who have had colds or bronchial conditions have leaned over a bowl of steaming water into which some eucalyptus essential oil has been dropped. With their eyes shut and their heads covered by a towel or some other covering, they have inhaled the essential oil vapors deeply

[4]Dr. Alan R. Hirsch, M.D., PACP, Neurologic Director, Smell & Taste Treatment and Research Foundation, Chicago, Illinois 60611.

through the nose. The volatile molecules of that euca-lyptus may be absorbed into the bloodstream via the absorbent mucus membrane of the nasal cavity, or the bronchial tract, or the lung. It is still the mechanism of smell, but it is also an absorption method into the body.

The aroma aspect of essential oils is very impor-tant. It is remarkable that our sense of smell is so com-plex and able. It is also interesting that we are drawn by sweet aroma to the very things which do us good. Some would see that as a reason to avoid them, as if it is child-like and naive to assume that if it smells good, it is good. Others would say this is God's work — drawing us towards the land's goodness, the profound gift. The mystery remains — why should most essen-tial oils smell so good?

Essential oils should not be underestimated. These sweet-smelling molecules float through the air like angels but they also deter bacteria, viruses, and fungi, and they make us feel good emotionally. Can we afford to be without them?

Percutaneous Absorption

It is a fact that essential oils are absorbed through the skin and it is easy to test this. Take a small smear of lavender oil and put it on your cheek. Pretty soon you will feel the lavender in your mouth and have the dis-tinct impression that the lavender molecules have actually passed through your flesh. For a more impres-sive result, put a dab of garlic oil on your foot and wait for the aroma to appear on your breath. Then ask yourself, how did the essential oil molecules travel through your body so fast? It's a question that science is not yet able to answer.

From a basic structural point of view, there is very little difference between people and essential oils. We are made of — more or less — the same stuff because we have the same evolutionary history. This may explain why essential oils seem to move through the body with such ease. Clearly, many essential oil molecules pass through the epidermis and enter the body, as can be seen when components of the essential oil are recovered from blood after being applied in a massage oil. It is also possible that because the molecules are so small they simply travel via the interstitial fluid, which surrounds all cells, although it could also be that the essential oil molecules pass through the cells themselves.

The beauty of percutaneous absorption is that essential oils can be applied to that part of the body where the oil is required, or as near to it as possible. For example, ginger oil — which appears to be a great bone healer — can be applied directly to a broken toe. If the problem is an earache, ginger diluted in vegetable oil can be applied behind the ear and in a straight line down the neck over the clavicle, across the upper chest, and into the underarm. This could affect the lymphatic system, as well as the Eustachian tube. If the problem is a strained muscle, diluted ginger oil can be applied directly to that muscle.

The only areas of the body to which essential oils are never applied are the eyes and any of the delicate mucus membrane areas. In most other cases, the essential oil is first diluted in a vegetable "carrier" oil. The purpose of this is to allow the small amount of essential oil to be spread over a larger area. It appears that the molecules of vegetable oils are usually too large to pass through the epidermis; the carrier simply allows the essential oil to be spread in the small volumes that are required. Sometimes, in special circumstances, essential oils are applied neat (undiluted) — as in the case of lavender for burns, or to treat insect bites.

Antibiotic, Anti-viral, and Anti-fungal Properties of Essential Oils

In some respects it is easy to see how essential oils work. For instance, the oil of thyme has been shown in many laboratory tests to be an extremely powerful antibiotic agent due to the activity of certain chemical components such as thymol. Therefore, it comes as no great surprise that most bacterial infections clear up when an antibiotic essential massage oil, such as thyme diluted in vegetable oil, is rubbed on the chest.

The antibiotic and other anti-microbial properties of essential oils have especially been researched in France, where aromatherapy has traditionally been employed more for infection control than anything else. This emphasis may have to do with the fact that in France, to be an "aromatherapist," you first have to be qualified as a physician, a profession which obviously has to deal with a great number of infections.

It is not so strange that the sweet-smelling essential oils should have powerful anti-microbial actions. After all, plants have to deal with invading bacteria, fungi, and viruses, just as people do, and over the millennia some plants have developed the capacity to fight them quite effectively. When certain essential oils are tested in the laboratory, it's clear that antibacterial action occurs, which makes us wonder whether essential oils contain the plant's immune system, or defense mechanism, in liquid form. This is not to say that all essential oil-producing plants have a disease-free existence; they may each have developed mechanisms for in fighting *particular* organisms. By understanding the individual germ-fighting profiles of each essential oil, we can best chose which to use for our own particular situation.

Around the world today, a lot of research is being carried out on the antibiotic, anti-viral, and anti-fungal action of essential oils. The third world in particular is concerned with developing anti-microbial substances which can be produced efficiently on home soil. In particular, exciting work with natural essences has been carried out in Egypt, India, and Zimbabwe. The benefits to such nations now conducting research into essential oils is two-fold. Not only can growing these products provide useful essential oils for the producer nation, it also provides a new cash crop to sell for foreign exchange by supplying the growing international aromatherapy market. The developed world has, in recent years, concentrated its research efforts into man-made chemical substitutes. Over the past seventy years a vast amount of scientific knowledge on essential oils has been accumulated in the USA, Britain, France, Australia, Russia, Poland, Hungary, Switzerland, and elsewhere. This information continues to be built upon, and becomes more urgent as bacteria and other microbes develop resistance to today's commonly-used medicines.

Cleansing Action

Those of us who work with essential oils on a daily basis can see their cleansing action quite clearly when used for skin care and for treatment of cellulite. If the correct oils are applied, certain toxins appear to be cleared from the body and the results are soon apparent. What seems to happen is that the toxins, the free-radicals, cell debris, heavy metals, renegade cells, fungi, bacteria, viruses, or other debris, may become attached to the essential oils which are then excreted from the body in the usual ways. The essential oils could be seen as rubbish collectors, attaching themselves to the unwanted agents and taking them to the exits for disposal.

Natural Balance

Essential oils seem to have the effect of bringing balance to the human organism. This is understandable because certain essential oils are thought to have "phytohormones" — molecules that mimic some of the hormones naturally occurring in the human body —

acting as messengers, or keys, for the related system. Other essential oils are "adaptogens" — they work at balancing the sympathetic nervous system. This means that the essential oil will respond to the body's requirements at any given time. If the system is stimulated and needs relaxing, the essential oil will do that, but if the system is sluggish, the oil will stimulate it. This may seem paradoxical at first but not if one has a basic belief in the wisdom of the body being able to take from the environment that which can do it the most good.

The Mind/Body/Spirit Connection

The spiritual dimension of essential oils is well known and has been used by people throughout recorded history. Indeed, from the earliest times it is clear that people have been using essential oils — or the materials they are extracted from — in prayer, meditation, ritual, purification, and celebration. The association between aroma and spirituality is not simply aesthetic, but grows from the fact that people find themselves more easily able to experience the spiritual while certain aromas are being used. The aroma seems to facilitate a connection with the spiritual dimension, making it a sort of highway to the soul.

People are a physical/mental/spiritual complex, and essential oils seem to have the ability to work on all three at the same time in some cases, or at least act as links between aspects of the self bringing the whole into balance. There is no way to prove this point experimentally; I am simply describing an experiential phenomenon which people appreciate. "Wholeness" is not scientifically quantifiable, but is no less real.

Synergy

Each essential oil is made up of dozens, if not hundreds, of components. These act not only in synergy with each other, giving the individual essential oil a particular characteristic and efficacy, but when you blend two or more essential oils together, you create another much more complex synergistic effect. Even blending one drop of (a) and two drops of (b) gives a different effect than two drops of (a) and one drop of (b). Aromatherapists marvel at the complexity of the system, and appreciate its effects. Synergy is basically the rule that the whole is more than the sum of the parts, and blends of essential oils working well together seem to enhance each other's effectiveness. This blending is a skill which is acquired with time and experience.

Chapter 3

How Essential Oils Are Used

*E*ssential oils are extremely versatile to use. The best-known method involves combining one or more essential oils with a vegetable base or carrier oil to make a "massage oil." Aromatherapists use these for medicinal or therapeutic purposes and usually apply them with massage. However, a massage oil can also simply be applied to the body, as one would apply any body oil, lotion, or cream. Aestheticians use essential oil massage oils to improve skin tone. At home, essential oils can be used in both these ways, but all this is just the tip of the iceberg because essential oils can be used in literally dozens of ways.

Because certain essential oils have antiseptic properties, they can be added to warm water and used as a kitchen or bathroom surface wipe. This simple procedure works well in most situations and housework is made that much easier by knowing you are not using man-made products that damage the environment. Plus, of course, essential oils smell wonderful . . . and that's not all. Use lavender to uplift the spirit — and heal cuts on your hands! Geranium, meanwhile, will ease the soul — while helping the circulation! Essential oil air fresheners are easily made by adding them to a clean plant sprayer which is half-full of warm water. To make clothes smell fresh, put a couple of drops of your favorite essential oil onto a cotton-wool ball or tissue and place it in wardrobes or drawers. Lavender has the added advantage of deterring moths.

Office workers also appreciate essential oils. In the morning, there is nothing to give you a zip like a shower using a drop of grapefruit essential oil on your washcloth. I feel wide awake just thinking about it! For a job interview, there is nothing to touch bergamot — which gives quiet, cool confidence, while for the efficient working of the brain, basil is the thing. It is not always possible to use a diffuser in the workplace, even if it is the portable variety which requires no flame or electricity to activate the aromatic volatile molecules within the essential oils.[5]

However, this isn't a problem. You can take a small bottle of your chosen essential oil or mix of oils to work, and simply inhale deeply from it. Or just put

---

[5]This refers to the Landel diffuser, avaliable from Essentially Yours — see "Suppliers" appendix in back of book.

some on a tissue before leaving for work and sniff from it when you feel the need. After lunch, a nice uplifting blend of lemon and rosemary will get you through the afternoon alert, efficient, and calm.

To keep bugs at bay, some people also put neat essential oil on their clothes — on socks and collars, for example, to keep mosquitoes away (they can't stand the smell of lavender). If you do get stung by a mosquito, ant, or bee, one smear of lavender oil will ease the pain and ensure quick healing. Or the essential oil, peppermint for example, can be placed neat around doors to keep mice out. Travelers also appreciate the fact that certain oils seem to repel insects, and a few drops on strange beds can prevent bites from unwelcome creatures which may be living there. Even public sinks and toilet seats can be wiped with a tissue that's got a few drops of antibiotic essential oil on it — a simple procedure that offers considerable comfort of mind.

More commonly, essential oils are used in the bathtub — four to six neat drops on the surface of the water after it's been run. Just swish the water and oil around and step in, lie back, and relax. They say that good things come in small packages and with essential oils that is certainly true! For tired feet, a few drops of essential oil in a foot bath seems nothing short of a miracle. Essential oils have been traditionally used by our grandparents in steam inhalations — eucalyptus in the case of colds being a common example. Just place the oil on the surface of a bowl of steaming water, cover the head with a towel, and inhale. And a few drops of any essential oil can similarly be put on a bowl of steaming water, and left on the floor by the bed overnight.

Essential oils are so versatile because they are highly concentrated. In many instances, all that's required is one drop. They can be purchased in small bottles, about the size of a lipstick and easily portable. Essential oils can literally be used anywhere. They can be diffused in the atmosphere, or applied directly to the skin in the form of massage oil, and used with water, in various ways, and in some cases, even used neat — i.e., undiluted. As we shall see, there are many variations on these basic themes and later in this section I provide a guide to the quantities of essential oil to use with each of the various methods of use.

*W*hat is Aromatherapy?

Simply put, aromatherapy is the therapeutic use of natural aromatic substances — essential oils. The "aroma" in "aromatherapy" refers to the fact that all essential oils have a characteristic smell, while the "therapy" refers to the fact that these oils are used for healing. This "therapy" aspect has several branches. Of course, people have always used pleasant aromas to cheer themselves up, as women do when they apply perfume. We find perfume uplifting and it somehow forms a character into which we fit ourselves. Perfume in the form of incense has also traditionally been used in religious contexts because it is known to uplift the spirit. People have preferences in both perfume and incense. Some find aromas particularly helpful in a strange, almost inexplicable, way. We now know, through scientific experimentation, that aromas exert an influence on the brain, and pictures of brain scans show this process at work.

Aromatherapy gained its popularity as an easy and natural method of stress relief. Certain essential oils, either applied in a massage, in bathtubs, or diffused in the atmosphere, make people feel more relaxed and confident. As mentioned earlier, this aspect of aromatherapy has gained scientific credence over recent years and today, especially in Japan, banks and other large companies use essential oils diffused in the atmosphere to make their customers feel comfortable and relaxed in their offices or shops.

Historic research shows that people have been using essential oils, or their forerunners — unguents, — as medicine for as long as we know. Indeed, without natural plant products in ancient times, there wouldn't have been any medicine! Today's plants are just as good for us as they have ever been, so long as they have not been damaged by chemical pollutants. They haven't suddenly stopped being medicines just because chemical replacements have been invented! Most of the research on essential oils concentrates on their medicinal qualities. It is these qualities which interest the doctors, paramedics, and nurses who, in increasing numbers, use essential oils as an adjunct to their work. In Britain, essential oils are being used in many hospital contexts, from labor rooms in maternity wards to intensive care units, and aromatherapy is increasingly available through the public health care system.

Hospices also find essential oils extremely helpful. For example, at the London Lighthouse, a specialist facility for the care of people with AIDS, aromatherapy is the most requested service that they offer.

"Aromatherapy" also refers to the use of essential oils for beauty and body care treatments. In this context, aromatherapy is one of the most popular treatments around the world, with clinics all over Europe specializing in techniques which employ essential oils. Essential oils are extremely effective for cellulite reduction, which is a detoxification procedure, and because some essential oils can quicken the production of body cells, they are often used in beauty-care revitalization treatments. Indeed, commercial product manufacturers are so aware of the beneficial qualities of essential oils they make sure to advertise that they are used in their preparations. However, as we shall see later, from a legal point of view there is no difference between an "essential oil" which is the pure extract of the named plant — what you and I understand as an essential oil — and a chemical copy. For this reason many commercial preparations which call themselves "aromatherapy" products have nothing whatsoever to do with the pure plant essences we know and love. By using the word "aromatherapy" in a context it does not belong, unscrupulous companies are cashing in on the fact that essential oils are known to work, and that people prefer the goods they use to be natural and pure.

Likewise, the word "aromatherapist" can be very misleading. It can refer both to someone who has attended a two or four year fully-comprehensive training program, and to someone who has merely attended a weekend introductory home-use course. In Britain and Europe, there is a good system of training and qualification which gives graduates the right to call themselves "an aromatherapist," and advertise their qualifications by using initials after their names. In particular, respect is given to those who are members of the International Federation of Aromatherapists (MIFA Reg.), members of the Register of Qualified Aromatherapists (MRQA), or International Society of Professional Aromatherapists (ISPA). Aromatherapy is relatively new in America and Canada so similar professional organizations are not as active. A new organization, however, the National Association for Holistic Aromatherapy, has now been set up to coordinate the profession within the United States, and Canadian aromatherapists are currently in the process of forming their own professional body.

Home Use

Essential oils can be very effective when used at home, just as they are when used by a therapist. There are many useful massage books on the market, written for the layperson and including self-massage. However, home use isn't limited to massage. There are many other effective methods of use which are simple and easy — and fun!

Aside from the methods listed with the recommended quantities later in this book, essential oils can be incorporated into all kinds of items and given as presents to family and friends. A homemade essential oil pomander for use with clothes hangers brings pure delight, while candles made using your favorite essential oils guarantee that you can always have that particular aroma around you when desired. Note paper and envelopes absorb the aroma of essential oils very well and all you have to do is place one or two drops on a tissue and place that in the box or container. After a few days, the paper will take on the aroma you have chosen and your correspondents will now have, besides your written message, an aromatic reminder of you! Such is the pleasure of aromatherapy.

One of the most cherished and appreciated aspects of essential oil use at home is the fact that it gives you a great deal more control over your life. Health is, of course, the greatest gift and essential oils are primarily about maintaining good health and well-being. Imagine how marvelous it is to be able to do something positive and effective when a member of the family is struck down with the flu, a cold or cough, by an infection, or by sprains and muscular aches. Many common ailments are easily dealt with by using essential oils. You will wonder how you ever managed before!

Another great benefit of using essential oils at home as a first-aid measure is that you can deal with a problem immediately. If a child wakes with an earache at three o'clock in the morning, you can deal with it there and then. If, in the early evening, your baby has colic and is crying constantly, the doctor's office is closed and you are at your wit's end, just five drops of dill essential oil diluted in 30 mls (1 oz) vegetable oil

— of which you use just a few drops — will help solve the problem. It is precisely because essential oils are so practical that people all over the world turn to them in times of difficulty, as you would turn to a reliable and competent friend. Of course, even the best of friends cannot be expected to do everything and sometimes professional help will be needed.

Aside from the considerable benefits in terms of well-being, using essential oils is like taking a bit of nature and bringing it into the house. We all need this desperately, especially if we live in cities. Few of us can now, as our ancestors did, walk through the fields and inhale the life-giving fragrance produced by flowers, plants, and trees. Such simple and beneficial delights, like the natural environment we evolved with, are mostly gone. (At least they are rare in most residential and working areas.) Most of us go through our day completely devoid of the goodness provided by nature. Yet we yearn for it, we need it, as a flower needs the sun. When you use essential oils, however, this yearning can be satisfied. Nature can be brought indoors, where we live and breathe, in the purest, most concentrated form — essential oils — and made a daily part of our lives. Using essential oils at home is easy, beneficial, and just plain nice!

Special Treatments

Certain groups of people are advised to use caution with essential oils. These are: babies, children, pregnant women, people suffering pain because of long-term medical conditions, the terminally ill, people who are taking large quantities of tranquilizers, those addicted to alcohol, and those addicted to substances known as "street drugs," or abusers of same. These are considered special cases and the dosages vary according to the condition. To use essential oils for these conditions, please refer to the "Special Treatments" section that follows the "General Guidelines" chart. It outlines these special cases, and details which essential oils are contraindicated or should be avoided altogether.

Base Oils

"Base" oils are vegetable oils that act as carriers for essential oils, allowing the very small molecules of essential oils to be spread over a larger area of skin. These base or carrier oils also prevent skin from absorbing too much essential oil at any given time, depending on the weight or thickness of the carrier oil being used. The thicker the carrier oil, the less essential oil is absorbed by the skin, and the thinner the carrier oil, the more essential oil is absorbed.

As often as possible, the base oils should be organic (grown without pesticides, etc.) and cold-pressed (extracted without the use of heat). Certain carrier oils act far better with essential oils than others. For example, olive oil is not used at all in traditional aromatherapy. Others, such as jojoba nut oil and avocado oil, although classified as vegetable or nut oils, are not used on their own because they are just too heavy. Instead, small quantities of these are blended with other carrier oils so their skin-nourishing properties can be taken advantage of.

Recommended Base Oils

Almond oil, apricot kernel oil, peach kernel oil,
hazelnut oil, grapeseed oil, camellia oil,
macadamia oil, coconut oil

The choice of base oil depends a great deal on the particular properties of that oil. Likewise, certain other vegetable or nut oils have properties which are useful in particular situations. Here are some particularly good mixers:

Good Mixers

Wheat germ oil, rose hip seed oil, borage oil, carrot oil,
evening primrose oil, avocado oil, jojoba oil

Blending

As mentioned previously, base oils can be used individually or blended together to create a base oil particular to your own skin type and therapeutic requirements. The basic rule to follow is to always put the larger amounts into the bottle first, adding the other ingredients of your blend in order of greatest volume. Then put the top on the bottle and roll it vigorously between the palms of your hands, allowing the molecules of all the base oils to become well blended. The following suggestions for base oil can be used for any essential oil formula, whether for medical or beauty purposes:

Revitalizing Body Carrier Oil

10 mls ($\frac{1}{3}$ oz) almond oil, 10 mls ($\frac{1}{3}$ oz) apricot kernel oil, 5 mls (100 drops or $\frac{1}{6}$ oz) macadamia oil, 5 mls (100 drops or $\frac{1}{6}$ oz) grapeseed oil, 4 drops of carrot oil, and 4 drops of jojoba oil

---

Revitalizing Face Carrier Oil (any skin type)
15 mls (½ oz) camellia oil, 10 mls (200 drops or ⅓ oz)
almond oil, 3 mls (60 drops or ⅒ oz) macadamia oil,
1ml (20 drops) rose hip seed oil, 1 ml (20 drops)
avocado oil, and 2 drops of borage oil

---

*G*eneral Guidelines for Self-Use
A-to-Z Reference of Essential Oil Applications

HOW TO USE	AMOUNT TO USE
BATH	**Up to 8 drops**

Run the bath as usual, then add the drops of essential oil and swish the water around. Keep the bathroom door closed to keep the aroma in the room. Essential oils can be used in their concentrated form or diluted in a small amount of vegetable oil, milk, or milk powder. Diluted essential oils used in the bath are gentler to sensitive skin.

HOW TO USE	AMOUNT TO USE
CLOTHING	**1 or 2 drops**

Most essential oils will leave a mark on clothes so only use this method if absolutely necessary, and on clothes you are prepared to see damaged. This is useful when in areas where there are many insects, especially midges and mosquitoes. Put the essential oil on socks or shoes, on the bottom of shorts or trouser legs, or on the collar, sleeves, or cuff of shirts, etc. To keep insects away from your head, wear a hair band or scarf and apply the oil there.

It's also useful for students who want to inhale a concentration-enhancing aroma when they're taking an exam to put it on the edge of the cuff and pretend to be rubbing an itchy nose!

HOW TO USE	AMOUNT TO USE
COMPRESS	3 to 5 drops

There are two methods that can be used with compresses. Always use 100% natural material, unbleached if possible. Compresses can be used hot or cold.
1) Place the essential oil in half a cup of water, dampen the compress in the cup, and place over the problematic area.
2) Wet the compress, and then apply the essential oil to the wet material.

HOW TO USE	AMOUNT TO USE
COTTON BUD	1 or 2 drops

Put the undiluted essential oil onto the cotton bud and apply directly to the affected area.

HOW TO USE	AMOUNT TO USE
DIFFUSER	As desired

There are a wide range of diffusers available on the market, mostly of the pottery type or electrical bowl type. Both of these rely on heat to activate the molecules of the essential oil, making them more volatile. It is important to keep water in the bowl, or the essential oil will burn. Also, the bowl should be non-porous and cleaned between each blend of essential oils that is used.

The new diffuser which uses no heat has a specially designed filter. It resembles a small lamp and can be safely used in all situations. It is also easily portable.

Nebulisers or oil vaporizers which issue a fine spray of essential oil into the atmosphere were designed for clinical use. They should not be used at home as the quantities of essential oil consumed can be too high and easily damage furnishings and paintings and are often difficult to clean between each different blend of essential oils.

HOW TO USE	AMOUNT TO USE
DRESSING	**1 to 2 drops applied directly onto a dressing**

This method is used to help stop the spread of infection and to promote wound healing. Put the essential oil directly onto the dressing that will cover the affected area — such as Band-Aids (the fabric part), bandage, lint, cotton. If the area is already dressed, put the essential oil on the external surface, provided the dressing surface is a material and not a plastic.

HOW TO USE	AMOUNT TO USE
FACE MASK	**1 drop per 10 mls ($\frac{1}{3}$ oz) of face mask**

Essential oils can be added to any natural face mask. The essential oil should be chosen depending on your skin type and the action on the skin you want it to achieve — as a treatment for acne, as a general stimulant, as a cleanser, as a purifier, rejuvenator, etc.

HOW TO USE	AMOUNT TO USE
FACE OIL	**2 to 15 drops in 30 mls (1 oz)**

Use the same method as making a massage oil for the body. However, use a more skin-nourishing carrier or base oil with additional nut or seed oils depending on the skin type.

HOW TO USE	AMOUNT TO USE
FACE TONIC	**1 to 5 drops in 100 mls (3 $\frac{1}{3}$ oz) water**

Boil either mineral or distilled water. While it's still hot add the essential oil and shake vigorously to combine. Then pour through an unbleached coffee filter and bottle. Leave to cool before using.

Hydrolats (a water by-product of essential oil production) can also be used either diluted by 50% or used as purchased.

HOW TO USE	AMOUNT TO USE
FOOT BATH	**5 drops in a bowl of water**

Fill a large bowl with warm water and add the essential oil, swishing it around. For a really relaxing foot bath, place some round smooth pebbles in the bottom of the bowl and rub the feet gently back and forth over them.

HOW TO USE	AMOUNT TO USE
FRICTION	**10 to 30 drops to 30 mls (1 oz) alcohol**

Friction is a term that is often used to describe the action of rubbing a part of the body, usually utilized by sports therapists.

Add the essential oil to ethyl alcohol (also known as rubbing alcohol) and shake well each time before use. Can be used all over the body but not on the face or delicate mucus membrane areas.

HOW TO USE	AMOUNT TO USE
GARDENING	**4 to 8 drops in a gallon of water**

Certain essential oils can be very effective as plant misters for microbial infection or used as an insect deterrent on plants. Add the essential oil to water and leave to blend for 24 hours. The most effective essential oils for gardening seem to be those extracted from trees, such as tea tree. Essential oils should never be combined with chemical gardening products but can be used with other natural organic methods.

HOW TO USE	AMOUNT TO USE
GARGLE	**1 to 2 drops per 30 mls (1 oz) of water**

First, thoroughly mix the essential oil in a teaspoon of honey. Then dilute with warm water until the honey is thoroughly dissolved. Then gargle with a small amount of the mixture and spit out. Do not swallow.

HOW TO USE	AMOUNT TO USE
GAUZE	**1 to 2 drops**

Put the undiluted essential oil on the gauze before applying over the affected area.

HOW TO USE	AMOUNT TO USE
HIGH DILUTION	**1 drop of essential oil to 3 drops of vegetable oil**

Used in cases of acute infection, where a high concentration of essential oil is required but where neat essential oil cannot be used because of excessive skin dryness, for example, or when the area cannot be massaged because of the risk of spreading infection.

   Simply dab onto the affected area. Should not be used for longer than seven days. Only use with those essential oils directed by the HDIL instruction given in Chapter 6. Do not exceed recommended dosage.

HOW TO USE	AMOUNT TO USE
HOT TUB	**Up to a maximum of 15 drops**

Add the essential oil to the water, then swish it around. Essential oils are not water soluble and may leave a residue in or around any pipes.

HOW TO USE	AMOUNT TO USE
HUMIDIFIER	**Up to 8 drops per pint of water**

Add the essential oil to the water in the humidifier. If it's the type that hangs over radiators you don't have to worry about the essential oil making the apparatus sticky and dysfunctional. More complex machines, however, may be damaged by the sticky residue. Each humidifier should, therefore, be looked at individually for its ability to be used in conjunction with essential oils.

HOW TO USE	AMOUNT TO USE
INHALATION	**3 drops per bowl of water**

Put steaming water in a bowl and add the essential oil. Cover the head with a towel, which should be large enough to reach right down over the sides of the bowl with no space for fresh air to come in. Inhale the steam deeply through the nose. Always keep both eyes shut. Inhale for a few seconds then raise the towel so you can take a deep breath through the mouth, lower the towel, and inhale through the nose again.

HOW TO USE	AMOUNT TO USE
JACUZZI	**Up to a maximum of 15 drops**

Add the essential oil to the water, then swish it around. Essential oils are not water soluble and may leave a residue in or on pipes .

HOW TO USE	AMOUNT TO USE
LOTION & CREAM	**5 to 10 drops to each 30 mls (1 oz) of natural, unfragranced lotion or cream**

Use an unperfumed lotion or cream, made of natural ingredients. Add the required number of essential oil drops and mix well.

HOW TO USE	AMOUNT TO USE
MASSAGE OIL (for body)	**10 to 30 drops to each 30 mls (1 oz) vegetable (base or carrier) oil**

If using a single essential oil, add the essential oil to the base vegetable oil already in the bottle. If using a synergistic blend of essential oils, put the essential oils into the empty bottle first, mix well by rolling the bottle between the hands, then add the base vegetable oil.

To mix completely together, put the cap on the bottle, then roll between the palms of both hands, turn the bottle upside down a few times and repeat the rolling between hands.

HOW TO USE	AMOUNT TO USE
MEDICINE	As directed

Essential oils are used to treat many conditions, including those relating to the respiratory system, the reproductive system, the digestive system, circulatory system, and the nervous system, as well as for muscular disorders, first aid, and bacterial, fungal, and viral infections. They are also used to treat the psyche.

The methods used vary depending on the condition, the symptoms, whether acute or chronic, the age of the person, and the preferences and training of the practitioner.

HOW TO USE	AMOUNT TO USE
MOUTHWASH	10 to 15 drops in 100 mls (3 ½ oz) water

Use distilled or mineral water. Bring it to a boil, add the essential oil, stir vigorously, then pour the water through a coffee filter, preferably unbleached. Leave to cool, then bottle. Use as required.

HOW TO USE	AMOUNT TO USE
NEAT (undiluted)	1 to 2 drops

In some conditions, undiluted essential oils can be used due to the nature of the essential oil and the condition. For example, lavender oil works extremely well applied directly to the skin in the case of burns, but cannot be applied in a vegetable oil. Most conditions, however, do not require undiluted application. Also, some essential oils must not, due to their irritant potential, be applied undiluted to the skin.

In Chapter 6, "An A-to-Z Guide of Essential Oils Use," those conditions which respond to undiluted essential oil are clearly marked with "N," but only use this method with those oils recommended on the list.

Do not use this method for more than seven days.

HOW TO USE	AMOUNT TO USE
PERFUME	Up to 50% of the blend

Making perfumes is an art that takes many years to learn. However, some people have a favorite blend of essential oils they would like to use as a perfume. The essential oils can be diluted with an odor-free natural alcohol or an oil such as jojoba. Use a small amount from the bottle as you would a perfume. Avoid getting it on clothing.

HOW TO USE	AMOUNT TO USE
PILLOW	1 or 2 drops

Use essential oils on pillows to help breathing or sleeping. Simply put one or two drops of your chosen essential oil on the corner of your pillow (use an old pillowcase that you are not worried about damaging). Alternatively, put the essential oil on a cotton-wool ball and tuck it under the corner of the pillow, or inside the pillowcase. Avoid using on areas near the eyes.

HOW TO USE	AMOUNT TO USE
POTPOURRI	As desired

Add the essential oils to the potpourri in the same way as you would add a commercial synthetic potpourri-refresher product. Single essential oils or blends can be used.

HOW TO USE	AMOUNT TO USE
ROOM SPRAY	10 drops per half-pint of water

Use a new plant mister. Put warm water in the mister, add the essential oil, shake it vigorously, as essential oils are not water soluble, and then spray. Avoid spraying over fine furniture and fabrics and anything that could be damaged by water.

HOW TO USE	AMOUNT TO USE
RUB	**10 to 30 drops per each 30 mls (1 oz) vegetable oil or a natural spirit solution**

In this book, the term "rub" is distinct from using a massage oil — "rub" means simply to apply gently to the affected area without actually having to massage in any way.

HOW TO USE	AMOUNT TO USE
SAUNA & SWEAT LODGE	**Up to 5 drops maximum**

Mix the essential oil as best you can, in the water that is to be placed on the hot coals or rocks.

HOW TO USE	AMOUNT TO USE
SCALP TREATMENT	**2 to 3 drops in a carrier of 15 mls ($\frac{1}{2}$ oz)**

There are various base carriers that can be used for scalp treatments. These can include natural (botanical) ready-made scalp treatments to which you add the essential oils. Or the essential oil can be added to aloe vera gel, water, jojoba oil, and massaged into the scalp. Alternatively, simply add the essential oil to a bowl of final rinse water after washing your hair.

HOW TO USE	AMOUNT TO USE
SHAMPOO	**5 to 15 drops in 100 mls (3 $\frac{1}{3}$ oz)**

Essential oils can be added to any unperfumed shampoo which is made using natural ingredients. Mix well. Choose essential oils that can be used on sensitive skin.

HOW TO USE	AMOUNT TO USE
SHOWER	**1 to 2 drops**

Wash as usual. Then place the essential oil onto your wet washcloth and wipe over your body while the shower is running. Avoid delicate areas and use essential oils that can be used on sensitive skin.

HOW TO USE	AMOUNT TO USE
SILK FLOWER	**As desired**

Open the flower completely and place the essential oil right at the center. Close the flower again if desired. Remember that essential oils may cause discoloration so try this on one flower before proceeding with the others. Essential oils can also be placed on paper and put at the bottom of the vase.

HOW TO USE	AMOUNT TO USE
SITZ BATH	**2 to 3 drops per sitz bath**

A sitz bath is a bath in which you immerse only the lower half of your torso. The essential oils are added to the water and swished around well. The essential oils can be used undiluted or diluted in a small amount of vegetable oil, seaweed powder, milk, or milk powder.

HOW TO USE	AMOUNT TO USE
SPRAY Face & Body	**10 to 15 drops to each pint of water**

Add the essential oils to warm water, shake thoroughly, pour through a coffee filter, and place in a spray container. Useful for body or face.

HOW TO USE	AMOUNT TO USE
TISSUE or HANDKERCHIEF	**1 or 2 drops**

Simply put the essential oil onto a paper or fabric hand-kerchief and sniff from it when required.

HOW TO USE	AMOUNT TO USE
WASH	**20 to 30 drops in pint of warm water**

Mix the essential oils and water together in a bottle and shake well. Pour though a coffee filter and re-bottle. Useful for washing infected areas such as wounds, grazes, cuts, and for other body and facial treatments.

HOW TO USE	AMOUNT TO USE
WATER BOWL	**From 2 to 10 drops**

Boil a pint of water and put the steaming water in a heat-proof bowl, then add the essential oil. Place in an area of the room away from animals and children.

Special Treatments

SPECIAL CONSIDERATIONS	GENERAL DOSAGE RULES	SPECIAL NOTES
PREGNANCY	Cut all the suggested minimum-maximum dosages by half.	Certain essential oils should be avoided during pregnancy. The full list of these is in Chapter 5, "Precautions."
BABIES	For a massage oil, a total of: **newborn**: 1–3 drops in 2 oz or 60 mls vegetable oil. **2–12 mos**: 3–5 drops in vegetable oil. For all other methods use **a quarter** of the **minimum** quantities recommended. For baths, put the essential oil in a pint of warm water and pour through a coffee filter before adding to the bath.	Only use: **newborn**: chamomile roman, dill, lavender **2–12 mos**: as above plus mandarin, tangerine, eucalyptus radiata, tea tree
CHILDREN	For a massage oil, a total of: **1–5 yrs**: 5–10 drops diluted in 60 mls (2 oz) vegetable oil. **5–7 yrs**: 5–12 drops diluted in 60 mls (2 oz) vegetable oil. **7–12 yrs**: 5-15 drops diluted in 60 mls (2 oz) vegetable oil. For all	As indicated plus: **1–5 yrs**: geranium **5–7 yrs**: ginger, ravensara **7–12 yrs**: frankincense, cypress, rosemary, spearmint, lemon

SPECIAL CONSIDERATIONS	GENERAL DOSAGE RULES	SPECIAL NOTES
	other methods: **up to 7 years:** use **half** the **minimum** quantities recommended. **After 12 years:** use the minimum quantities. **For all ages:** use in the bath, put the essential oil in a pint of warm water and pour through a coffee filter before adding to the bath.	
CHRONIC PAIN	For a massage oil: 30 drops to 30 mls (1 oz) of vegetable oil. Other methods: up to maximum dosage.	Certain essential oils have analgesic properties. Look under "An A-to-Z Guide of Essential Oil Use," Chapter 6.
TERMINAL ILLNESS	During the last stages of terminal illness dosages should be half the recommended dosage.	Room fragrances are very helpful at this time, used in diffusers.
PEOPLE ON MEDICATION	For all methods use up to half the maximum recommended dosages. If using them as medicines, inform the physician. If using homeopathic medicines, inform the homeopath.	It is thought that essential oil use may negate the effect of homeopathy.

SPECIAL CONSIDERATIONS	GENERAL DOSAGE RULES	SPECIAL NOTES
RADIO-THERAPY TREATMENT	While undergoing radiotherapy essential oils should not be used during the treatment itself, but can be used in-between sessions to help alleviate soreness and radiation burns. Dosages should be half the maximum general dosage.	The only essential oils that should be used at this time until the treatments are completed are bio-wild (or organic) lavender (fresh flower, blue), chamomile roman, and tea tree.
PRE- & POST-OPERATIVE	In the **pre-operative** period the dosages should be half the maximum recommended and the physician should be informed if using essential oils for medicinal purposes. In the **post-operative** period essential oils can be used at maximum dosage if necessary to help lessen the risk of infection. If on medication, half the maximum general dosages should be used.	Certain essential oils can considerably lessen the risk of infection. These are lavender, tea tree, thyme linalol, ravensara, and eucalyptus radiata. They can be used post-operatively on the body and dropped directly onto the bedclothes. If diffused, however, stronger essential oils such as oregano, cinnamon, and red thyme can also be utilitized for infection control.

SPECIAL CONSIDERATIONS	GENERAL DOSAGE RULES	SPECIAL NOTES
TRANQUILIZER ADDICTION	During addiction all essential oil dosages should be half the maximum general dosage. Inform the physician that essential oils are being used.	While reducing the dosage of prescribed tranquilizers, essential oils that have a calming effect upon the nervous system should be used. See "An A-to-Z Guide of Essential Oil Use," Chapter 6, for guidance.
SUBSTANCE ADDICTION	During addiction all essential oil dosages should be half the maximum general dosage.	While reducing the dosage of addicted substance, essential oils that have a toning and purifying effect on the body should be used. See "An A-to-Z Guide of Essential Oil Use," Chapter 6, for guidance.
ALCOHOLISM	When using alcohol to excess all essential oil dosages should be half the maximum general dosage.	Essential oils that have a tranquilizing and purifying effect on the digestive and nervous system should be used. See "An A-to-Z Guide of Essential Oil Use," Chapter 6, for guidance.

In the above guidelines I have not mentioned the taking of essential oils orally (internally by mouth). Use of essential oils in this way should always be under the guidance of a qualified physician. In any case, this method is now thought to be the least effective way to use essential oils medicinally not only because it is subject to the digestive process, but because it is not as direct as the many other methods of using essential oils. Some practitioners, especially in France, still do prescribe essential oils to be taken in this way, but always in extremely low and precise dosages. They are given orally on a sugar lump or in a spoonful of honey, although most often they are diluted in some form of liquid to avoid irritation of the membranous lining of the esophagus. Mainstream medicine is now seeking other more effective ways of delivering medication which avoid using the digestive system, including the liver. For example, insulin in a crystallized form is being given to diabetics via inhalation.

For further information regarding the use of essential oils, please see Chapter 5, "Precautions."

*C*hapter 4

Buying and Storing Essential Oils

*B*uying essential oils is like buying anything else — you have to shop around. You may strike it lucky and quickly find the perfect vendor of essential oils. They should be supplied in dark bottles, with the Latin name available, if not on the bottle itself, then in the catalog. Also, the expiration date of the oil should be given on the bottle. Generally, oils last two years although citrus oils like lemon, for example, are said to have therapeutic vibrancy within them only for about six months, while others, such as eucalyptus, patchouli, frankincense, and sandalwood, retain their effectiveness for longer than the usual two years.

However, it is not a perfect world and to complicate things further, the term "essential oil" is legally used to describe all sorts of things which are not what you or I would expect — namely, a plant essence distilled from the plant named on the bottle. What happens is, to maximize profit, people sell bottles of liquid purporting to be "essential oil" when in fact it is a chemical construct made in a factory. This is legal, and a problem caused by the loose legal definition of "essential oil." Many so-called "aromatherapy" products are made using these man-made chemical materials. Another problem is that the bottle might quite correctly say "essential oil," because it does contain essential oils, but not the particular oil named on the label. In this case, wholesalers blend together essential oils which smell like the essential oil named on the label. This is done especially with the expensive essential oils like carnation — a fair copy of which can, by clever blending, be made using black pepper and ylang ylang or clove — all of which are much cheaper but can smell like carnation (to the inexperienced nose). Labels may also say the product inside is "pure" or "natural" — this is accurate but mis-leading because the substance inside the bottle is indeed natural, but not the natural substance the label leads you to believe it is. It may not be an essential oil at all, but a blend of other natural materials or natural chemicals designed to look like a particular essential oil, even when tested.

Those of us who use essential oils for professional therapeutic purposes need to know exactly where an essential oil is from because a lavender grown on the high Alps in France is different from one grown in China, for example, just as the clary sage grown in France has different properties than one grown in Russia. It is best not to buy oils which have been blended from different countries. We need to know exactly what we're buying and to this end some of us physically go to the growers themselves to make sure we know what that is. Obviously, the casual buyer cannot engage in this expense and trouble, and they should not need to if they are dealing with a reputable essential oil company. This brings us to the bottom line — how to establish which is and which is not a reputable company.

These are the things to watch out for:

1) If a whole range of essential oils is being sold at the same price in the same size of bottle, you can be absolutely sure the products inside do not accurately reflect what is on the label. On my current price list 10 milliliters (approximately 1/3 oz) of jasmine essential oil costs eighteen times as much as the same amount of grapefruit essential oil. *That's* how much essential oils can vary in price. Clearly, if a range is being sold all at the same price, something is wrong. It could be you are looking at man-made chemical constructs (and remember that the perfume industry has spent many years and many millions of dollars developing materials to mimic nature's smells). Alternatively, the essential oil could be diluted in a base or carrier oil, and should

be labeled accordingly.

2) Pure, undiluted essential oils should be sold in dark bottles, either brown, green, mauve, or blue, for example. If they are sold in clear glass bottles (or, even worse, clear plastic), the company isn't aware that this lets the light in and damages the goods — clearly a company to avoid.

3) Bottles should always have dropper tops which allow drops to be measured. This is a practical but more importantly a safety feature, so that if children happen to get their hands on the bottles and drink from them, they'll only consume a couple of drops before realizing that lemon essential oil is not lemonade! Also, essential oils evaporate and deteriorate when exposed to the air, and more air reaches the essential oil in bottles without dropper tops. Companies which sell essential oils without dropper tops should be avoided. Also, remember to always keep bottles out of the reach of children.

4) You should always be able to ascertain from the retailer the Latin name of the essential oil. Is the "eucalyptus," for example, eucalyptus globulus, eucalyptus citriodora, eucalyptus piperata, or eucalyptus radiata? These Latin names may not be on the label but the retailer should have a list somewhere that gives you that information. If he or she cannot provide you with the information because it has not been supplied to them, the

essential oil company should probably be avoided.

At this point you may think buying essential oils is too much trouble. But think of it like this: If you wanted to buy a car, you would not just go out and buy the first one you saw. You would speak to your friends who know something about cars, and ask their advice. So, ask friends, aromatherapists, or other health practitioners which companies they use. Find out where they are located and phone for a catalog or price list. Most essential oil companies have a mail-order service. Please see the end of this book for suppliers' addresses.

When you first begin to use essential oils, it may seem difficult to find the best suppliers. In time, however, your nose (which is the best guide to the subject — once trained with experience) will lead you on and teach you what to look for. As I said, buying essential oils is like buying anything else — shop around. Smell the oils, get familiar with the subject and, in time, you will locate a good supplier.

In Chapter 8, "Essential Oil Profiles," I have given some purchasing hints for each oil, in terms of color, viscosity, and smell. In general, although they are called "oils," essential oils are not in fact oily. If you were to put a seed oil, such as sunflower, on a piece of absorbent paper, the oil would sit there and still appear oily after a period of time. Essential oils are different. They soon evaporate, leaving no oily residue. It is somewhat more difficult to see this rule in operation with certain colored essential oils and absolutes which may leave an imprint of the color behind.

Containers and Storage

Essential oils should be kept in dark, glass bottles. The darkness is important to protect the contents from the sun's rays, while the alternative to glass — plastic — may fractionally dissolve, leaving microscopic particles in the essential oil. There is now a plastic on the market, called PET, which is biodegradeable and said not have this effect with essential oils, nor to emit pollutants or toxic gases when burned. This material is now being used by many aromatherapy companies. I wouldn't recommend using PET plastic for storing pure, undiluted essential oils, however it could be used for storing essential oils diluted in carrier vegetable oils.

Essential oils are volatile, which means they evaporate, so whatever container you use, ensure that the lid is kept tight at all times. Replace the lid immediately after using the essential oil or diluted oils. This will prevent not only evaporation but oxidation.

As far as is possible, essential oils and diluted oils should be kept in a cool, dark, dry place. Make sure there is no damp or direct heat in the area. For these reasons, bathrooms are not good places to keep them, because they get damp and hot. Keeping them in a cupboard in a cool room is ideal. Also, make sure they are out of reach of children.

Essential oils are flammable — they easily catch fire — so use caution. For example, if you wipe up some spilt essential oil with a tissue and place it in the garbage, it would be unwise to then dispose of an exhausted match in the same pail. Also, don't place a bin into which you have thrown tissues or other materials with essential oil on them in direct heat — near a sunny window for example — this may cause it to catch fire. Please be careful. Just remember, excessive heat and essential oils do not go together!

Solidification

Under cold conditions, some essential oils will crystallize and solidify. Rose otto and benzoin are classic examples of this. This effect does not hurt the essential oil nor affect its therapeutic ability. If the oil is placed in a warm room it will soon return to a fluid consistency. But never heat or boil the essential oil to quicken the process. If you are in a hurry, just hold the bottle in your warm hand for a few minutes, which will melt the essential oil just enough to produce the few precious drops you require right there and then.

Diluted Oils

If you make up a diluted essential oil — i.e., blend essential oils with a base vegetable oil — you should use it within six months. For this reason, when making up a diluted oil, always label it (saying what's in it, and who and what it is for) and include the date it was prepared. The natural preservative effect of essential oils may negate the need of using additives, but vegetable, nut, and seed oils go rancid and oxidize with age. As a result, they can smell rancid and may start to go cloudy. When this happens, it's time to discard the blend.

*C*hapter 5

PRECAUTIONS

*O*ne of the simplest safety precautions when using essential oils involves always washing your hands after mixing or applying them. This avoids the problem of later rubbing your eye, or another sensitive area of the body, such as a mucus membrane. Should essential oils be passed on from your hands to these more sensitive areas, it can result in a stinging sensation. And if essential oil gets into your eye it must be washed out immediately with cold sterile water.

*P*regnancy

Certain essential oils should be avoided during pregnancy and while breast feeding,

and these are listed below. There are no scientific studies reporting actual cases where either mother or fetus
have been harmed while using essential oils. Still, aromatherapists take the precautionary position that
some essential oils may contain components which
have a physiological action which could possibly have
a negative effect on pregnant women and thus their
avoidance is recommended. In particular, certain
essential oils may contain phytohormones, which
mimic the body's own hormones and thus have an
effect on the menstrual cycle. Clearly, during pregnancy, phytohormones are not required. Also, certain
essential oils which have a particularly powerful effect
on the central nervous system should be avoided.

Essential Oils Which Generally Should be Avoided During Pregnancy:

Basil, Cinnamon, Aniseed, Fennel, Juniper, Marjoram,
Rosemary, Thyme (Red and Linalol), Clary Sage, Oregano,
Clove, Nutmeg, Bay, Pimento Berry, Cistus, Hops, Sage,
Valerian, Spikenard, Black Pepper, Tarragon, Cedarwood,
Hyssop, Myrrh, Peppermint, Mace,
Cumin, Parsley Seed, Wintergreen, Birch

*Also refer to the list of essential oils which are
not safe to use in therapy by anyone,
and this is found at the end of this chapter.*

Aside from avoiding the essential oils listed above,
pregnant women are advised to use only half the usual
recommended minimum-maximum dose cited in
Chapter 3.

Skin can be especially sensitive during pregnancy.
Things you are never allergic to can now be found to
be allergenic and perfumes you previously loved can

now give you headaches or make you feel nauseous. Also, you may find yourself drawn to aromas you did not previously find appealing. All of this has to be taken into consideration so please smell the essential oil and see if your reaction to it has changed before using it. Another factor to consider is that during pregnancy it is fairly common for the woman's skin to experience temporary changes in pigmentation. For this reason, and because citrus essential oils can also cause this problem, they are only to be used for specific reasons and with caution. Also, read "Skin Sensitivity" below.

When the time comes for breast-feeding, make sure there is no oil whatsoever (either essential oil or base oil) on the nipple itself or on the area around it, against which the baby's cheek and head will be pressed. Also, continue to use the dosages for pregnancy, and continue to avoid the essential oils listed above. (There is one company I recommend which specializes in products for use during pregnancy, and this is listed under "Suppliers" in the Appendix.)

Skin Sensitivity

Skin is considered the largest organ of the body and to some degree, it reflects internal health. For example, toxins which have accumulated inside the body can be reflected externally on the skin as spots or rashes, while allergies to particular foods can be expressed on the surface of the skin as various types of marks — blotches, rashes, and so forth. Also, some viruses migrate to the skin — think about chicken pox which is contracted by airborne droplets but expressed on the skin as blisters and scabs.

Today many drugs are administered by stick-on patches applied to the skin. This happens with hormone replacement therapy (HRT), steroids, vitamins for people with an impaired digestive system, anti-smoking patches, slimming patches, etc. Also, allergies to foods, cosmetics, or petroleum products are ascertained by physicians testing on the skin. The allergic reaction may not affect the skin itself, but the skin is used as a diagnostic tool, a kind of mirror to internal goings-on. Thus, the skin has a two-way function in determining our health.

The skin can also have reactions to certain products, so most cosmetics come with the advice to "try on a small patch on the skin" before regular use. If you have any allergies to perfumes which may contain essential oils, it is wise to also test essential oils on a small patch of skin before using them more extensively. Simply put three drops in half a teaspoon of vegetable oil and use a small portion of this on a small area of skin. Wait for 24 hours to see if any reaction occurs. The same procedure applies if you are allergic to cosmetics, washing powders, or other products. The concentration of essential oils in perfumes is very low, so if you are allergic to perfumes it could be that you are actually allergic to one of the many petroleum-based products which are used in perfumes these days.

There are a great number of essential oils and clearly some people will be allergic to some of them, just as some people are allergic to certain foods or cosmetic products and perfumes. People who have an allergic reaction to citrus fruits should not use the citrus essential oils such as lemon, orange, mandarin, tangerine, yuzu, or lime — either on their own or in blends with other essential oils. Those with allergies to wheat should do a skin test before using wheat germ oil, sometimes used as a mixer in a base or carrier oil, although they may be allergic to the gluten in bread and not to wheat germ oil itself.

Using essential oils requires the use of common sense, and this is especially true if you have sensitive skin. The best course of action is to skin-test each essential oil before you use it, even if only using a small amount in blends. It is also important to use absolutely pure essential oils bought from reputable suppliers. There is great variation in the quality of essential oils available on the market. If you do have a reaction it may be because you are allergic, but it is also possible that you have bought a product which contains some synthetic chemical additives and that you may be having an allergic reaction to them. If skin sensitivity occurs, wash the area thoroughly and apply a soothing vegetable oil, such as almond.

Essential Oils to be Avoided by People with Sensitive Skin

Basil, Bay, Birch, Black Pepper, Cinnamon, Clove, Cumin, Fennel, Fir, Ginger, Lemon, Lemongrass, Lemon Verbena, Oregano, Parsley Seed, Peppermint, Pimento Berry, Pine, Tagetes, Red Thyme, Wintergreen

---

There are some essential oils which can have a

skin-irritating effect on some people, not necessarily those prone to skin sensitivity. These oils are listed below. In the case of lemon, problems are usually only caused when the product's shelf life has expired.

Essential Oils Which May be Skin Irritants for Some People

Basil, Benzoin, Birch, Black Pepper, Clove, Cinnamon, Ginger, Lemon, Lemongrass, Lemon Verbena, Oregano, Peppermint, Pimento Berry, Pine, Tagetes, Red Thyme, Wintergreen

---

Some essential oils cause photosensitivity, which means they increase the effect of the sun on the skin. These essential oils should not be used on any exposed areas of skin before going into the sunlight, especially by people with fair skin.

Essential Oils Not to be Used on the Skin Before Exposure to Sunlight

Angelica, Bergamot, Cumin, Grapefruit, Lemon, Lemon Verbena, Lime, Orange, Yuzu, Tangerine, Mandarin

---

Babies and Children

Not all essential oils are safe to use on babies and children. For a list of the essential oils which can be used safely, please see "Special Treatments" at the end of Chapter 3, which lists the oils that can be used for babies and children in various age groups. Recommended dosages are also given.

Contraindications

Please refer to the "Special Treatments" section at the end of Chapter 3. This section gives advice for people with chronic pain, terminal illness, those taking medication, receiving radiotherapy treatment, considering using essential oils either pre- or post-operatively, addicted to tranquilizers or alcohol, or abusing other substances.

In addition to the above conditions, there are certain situations which should be given special consideration before essential oils are used. These include the following:

Driving

If using essential oils to scent the car, avoid those that could make you feel so relaxed you are in danger of losing concentration. Avoid: benzoin, carnation, chamomile german, chamomile roman, geranium, hops, hyacinth, lavender, linden blossom, mace, marjoram, neroli, nutmeg, ormenis flower, petitgrain, rose maroc, sandalwood, spikenard, valerian, vetiver, and ylang ylang.

Epilepsy

The following essential oils should be avoided by those people prone to epileptic fits or those who may have a predisposition to epilepsy: fennel, hyssop, rosemary, sage, and wormwood.

Hypertension (High Blood Pressure)

It is recommended that people with high blood pressure avoid using the following essential oils: hyssop, rosemary, sage, and thyme.

Kidney and Liver Disease

People with kidney disease should avoid using fennel and juniper.

People with liver disease should avoid using essential oils altogether.

Furnishings and Clothing

Some essential oils will damage clothing or precious furniture if allowed to come into contact with them. In particular, velvet and silk are very delicate and can show marks easily — even if the mark is only made by water. Essential oils are liquid, and can likewise damage such materials. It is best to avoid using essential oils on or near any such sensitive materials used in clothing or furnishings. The air-diffusion method, which involves putting essential oils into a new plant mister with water and using as an air-freshener, should be used with care. The water in the spray can damage furnishings and polished furniture, as can the essential oils. Please do not use this method on or near such furnishings.

The citrus essential oils are very cleansing and are used as solvents in the computer industry and in effective hand-wash products designed to cut through stubborn grease. These essential oils should not be used near polished wooden furniture or near other furnishings which are liable to damage, or are particularly precious to you.

Fire Precautions

Essential oils are flammable. This means that they must be stored away from sunlight and other heat sources and care must be taken with the materials used with them, such as tissues used to mop up spills. See Chapter 4, "Buying and Storing Essential Oils."

Essential Oils Not to be Used Under Any Circumstances

The International Federation of Aromatherapists recommends that the following essential oils should not be used under any circumstances:

Bitter Almond	Rue
Boldo leaf	Sassafras
Calamus	Savin
Yellow Camphor	Southernwood
Horseradish	Tansy
Jaborandi leaf	Thuja
Mugwort	Wintergreen
Mustard	Wormseed
Pennyroyal	Wormwood

*C*hapter 6

An A-to-Z Guide of Essential Oil Use

*T*his chapter recommends essential oils to use for various situations, arranged in two sections: physical and emotional. There are often quite a few varieties of essential oils listed because in a clinical setting we are presented with individuals with very different symptoms, lifestyles, personalities, and problems. Therapists will look at an individual as a whole and need to be able to "throw the net wide," as it were, to give them the choice they need to deal effectively with each person. The general reader, however, doesn't need to employ this complexity of thought and so I have italicized the essential oils which are the generally most useful, and which can also be blended together well. The essential oils listed are those found within this book, having their own profiles in Chapter 8.

The material is arranged in alphabetical order, sometimes with sub-sections. In the right hand column you will find letters denoting a choice of different methods for using these essential oils. For details about quantities to use, and descriptions of the methods, see Chapter 3. A directory for the methods of use follows. The first entry, "A," if applicable, precedes the other methods because it is a direction as to how to use any of the following methods.

A	apply to the affected area directly, carefully and gently, without stimulating or moving it in any way.
B	bath
C	compress
CB	cotton bud
DS	dressing
FO	face oil
FB	foot bath
FM	face mask
FT	face tonic
G	gauze
GR	gargle
HDIL	high dilution
I	inhalation: various methods including water bowl, or inhalation directly from a tissue or bottle
LC	lotions and creams
M	massage
MW	mouthwash

N   neat

R   apply gently; see "Rub" in "Methods of Use"

RF   room fragrance: diffused into the atmosphere, by various room methods

S   spray

SB   sitz bath

ST   scalp treatment

W   wash

CONDITION	ESSENTIAL OILS	METHODS
ABDOMEN:		
bloated	*fennel,* cardamom, *peppermint*	R, M
wind	*fennel,* coriander, *peppermint*	R, M
colic (adult)	chamomile roman, *cardamom,* coriander, *peppermint,* fennel, ginger, juniper	R, M
pain	*black pepper,* eucalyptus radiata, lavender, fennel, ginger, cardamom, *peppermint,* ravensara	R, M, B
cramp	*black pepper,* chamomile roman, clary sage, coriander, lavender, *peppermint,* yuzu	R, M, B
ABSCESS, EXTERNAL: dry	*lavender,* manuka, ravensara, *tea tree*	A, G, C, N, R
weeping (with discharge)	bergamot, frankincense, *lavender,* manuka, *tea tree,* ravensara	A, G, C, N, W
breast	bergamot, *lavender,* manuka, *ravensara*	A, C, G, N, W, HDIL
ABSCESS, MOUTH:	manuka, *tea tree*	MW, CB
ABSCESS, DENTAL:	chamomile roman, chamomile german, manuka, *tea tree*	MW, CB
ACNE: general	benzoin, bergamot, cedarwood, chamomile german, eucalyptus radiata, geranium, grapefruit, juniper, *lavender,* lemon, lemongrass, litsea	FO, CB, S, W

CONDITION	ESSENTIAL OILS	METHODS
	cubeba, palmarosa, petitgrain, ravensara, *rosemary,* sandalwood, tea tree, thyme (see also "Skin Care")	
with redness	chamomile roman, chamomile german, *eucalyptus radiata,* geranium, juniper, *lavender*	FO, CB, S, W
pustule: (spots with pus)	bergamot, lemon, tea tree, *thyme linalol,* rosemary	FO, CB, S
scarring	benzoin, frankincense, *palmarosa, petitgrain*	FO, S, W
ADDICTION:	chamomile roman, clary sage, *bergamot,* jasmine, *juniper,* lavender, ylang ylang, yuzu	B, M, RF
ADENOIDS: enlarged	cypress, juniper, *eucalyptus* r*adiata, tea tree*	GR, MW, M (massage on the outside of the neck)
pus-covered	*clove,* eucalyptus radiata, manuka, *tea tree*	GR, MW, M
AGING: general	geranium, jasmine, ginger, *neroli, rose otto,* rosemary, thyme linalol, *yuzu* (see also "Skin Care, aging/mature")	M, B, R, I
ALLERGIES:	chamomile roman, *lavender,* rose otto	B, M, I, RF
ALOPECIA:	clary sage, *cypress,* ormenis flower, *rosemary,* thyme linalol	M, R, W
ANALGESIC: pain relief	black pepper, chamomile roman, *helichrysum,* yuzu	M, B, R, C, G
ANOREXIA: to relax	*bergamot,* chamomile roman, clary sage, lavender, *neroli,* palmarosa	B, M, I, RF
appetite stimulant	black pepper, cardamom, *coriander, fennel*	I, RF
strength-ening	cardamom, *ginger, lemon,* litsea cubeba, rosemary	I, RF, B, M
APHRODISIAC:	black pepper, cardamom, *jasmine,* neroli, rose otto, *rose maroc,* sandalwood, *ylang ylang*	M, B, RF

CONDITION	ESSENTIAL OILS	METHODS
APPETITE: lack of	basil, cardamom, *coriander*, *fennel*, rosemary	R, M, B, RF, I
loss of	chamomile roman, *coriander*, fennel, *ginger*, rosemary	R, M, B, RF, I
suppressed	*cinnamon*, *clove*, fennel, ginger	RF, I
ARTHRITIS: general	benzoin, *black pepper*, cedarwood, chamomile german, chamomile roman, cinnamon, cypress, ginger, *helichrysum*, juniper, lavender, lemon, eucalyptus radiata, eucalyptus globulus, *marjoram*, oregano, *rosemary*, tea tree, thyme linalol	M, R, C, B
redness (with heat)	*chamomile roman*, chamomile german, juniper, *lavender*	M, R, C, B
swelling	*cypress*, *juniper*, lavender	M, R, C, B
pain	benzoin, *black pepper*, chamomile roman, cypress, ginger, *helichrysum*, lavender, rosemary	M, R, C, B
ASTHMA:	cedarwood, chamomile german, cypress, eucalyptus globulus *eucalyptus radiata*, eucalyptus citriodora, frankincense, lavender, *marjoram*, neroli, pine, rose otto, yuzu	M, R, B, I, RF
ATHLETE'S FOOT:	lavender, *manuka*, myrrh, palmarosa, patchouli, *tagetes*, tea tree	FB, N, CB
BABIES: colic	lavender, *chamomile roman*	M, R
colds & coughs	eucalyptus radiata, frankincense, *tea tree*	M, R (chest and neck) B, RF
cradle cap	*lavender*, tea tree	M, R
earache	*chamomile roman*, tea tree	M, R (down neck and around jaw bone)
minor discomforts	lavender, *chamomile roman*, mandarin	M, R, B
diaper rash	chamomile roman, *lavender*,	C, G, B, R,

CONDITION	ESSENTIAL OILS	METHODS
	manuka, tea tree	HDIL
sleeplessness	*chamomile roman*, lavender, neroli	RF, M, R, B
teething	*chamomile roman*	R, M
		(outer jaw massage)
BABY BLUES: (post-natal depression)	benzoin, *bergamot*, chamomile roman, jasmine, *neroli*, linden blossom, rose otto, *rose maroc*, yuzu	B, M, R, RF, FO, S
BACK PAIN:	*basil*, black pepper, chamomile roman, clary sage, cypress, ginger, *helichrysum*, marjoram, oregano, peppermint, rosemary, spikenard, thyme	M, B, R
BACTERIAL INFECTION:	(see "Antibiotic Essential Oils" list in Chapter 8)	
BALDNESS:	lavender, *litsea cubeba*, *jojoba*, *rosemary*, cypress	M, ST
BED SORES:	bergamot, *lavender*, frankincense, *manuka*, ravensara, *tea tree*, yuzu	A, C, G CB, HDIL
BED WETTING: (associated with stress)	chamomile roman, lavender, *mandarin, petitgrain*	B, M, RF
BELCHING:	cardamom, coriander, *fennel*, ginger	I, M, RF
BILIOUSNESS:	basil, black pepper, ginger, lemon, marjoram, *peppermint*	I, M, R
BITES: animal	bergamot, lavender, lemon, manuka, oregano, helichrysum, *tea tree, thyme (linalol* or *red)*	A, N, CB G, W, DS HDIL
insect	eucalyptus globulus, eucalyptus radiata, *lavender*, lemon, manuka, patchouli, *tea tree*	A, N, CB, G, W, DS
human	bergamot, *lavender*, helichrysum, oregano, tea tree, *thyme linalol*	A, N, CB G, W, DS
reptile	clove, *lavender*, oregano, tea tree, *thyme (linalol* or *red)*	A, N, CB G, W, DS
BLACK EYE:	*lavender*	C
BLADDER INFECTION:	*sandalwood*, tea tree	B, SB, M
	(see also "Antibiotic Essential Oils" list in Chapter 8)	

CONDITION	ESSENTIAL OILS	METHODS
BLISTERS:	*benzoin, geranium, lavender,* myrrh, tagetes, tea tree, yuzu	C, DS, G, CB
BODY ODOR:	bergamot, clary sage, *cypress,* geranium, juniper, *lemon*	R, B, M, S, W
BOILS:	*bergamot,* chamomile german, lavender, juniper, lemon, litsea cubeba, tea tree, thyme linalol, *ravensara,* yuzu	C, G, W, N, CB, HDIL
BOWEL DISORDERS: with inflammation	chamomile roman, chamomile german, cypress, *lavender,* litsea cubeba, patchouli, *peppermint*	M, R, C, B
with pain	cypress, fennel, *helichrysum, peppermint*	M, R, C, B
with discomfort	helichrysum, *patchouli, peppermint*	M, R, C, B
with swelling	cypress, *fennel, juniper*	M, R, C, B
BREATH, BAD:	*clove,* lavender, *peppermint,* tea tree (see also "Gum Infections")	MW, G
BREATHING DIFFICULTIES:	cedarwood, eucalyptus globulus, eucalyptus radiata, *pine,* ravensara	I, B, M, R
BRONCHITIS: general	basil, benzoin, cedarwood, clove, eucalyptus citriodora, eucalyptus globulus, *eucalyptus radiata,* frankincense, marjoram, myrrh, oregano, pine, sandalwood, *ravensara,* rosemary, tea tree, thyme (red and linalol)	I, B, RF, M, R
acute	*cinnamon,* eucalyptus globulus, ravensara, thyme (red)	I, B, RF, M, R
chronic	benzoin, eucalyptus radiata, *pine, ravensara*	I, B, RF, M, R
with cough	*benzoin, cypress,* ravensara, sandalwood	I, B, RF, M, R
with congestion	*eucalyptus globulus,* eucalyptus radiata, frankincense, helichrysum, tea tree, thyme, *ravensara*	I, B, RF, M, R
BRONCHI-OLOTIS:	cinnamon, *pine, ravensara,* thyme linalol	I, M, R, B

CONDITION	ESSENTIAL OILS	METHODS
BRUISES:	lavender, fennel, geranium, *helichrysum, ormenis flower,* rosemary, tea tree	N, C, G, DS
BUNIONS:	*chamomile german,* marjoram, peppermint, *tagetes*	CB, M, R, FB
BURNS: (first degree)	*lavender* (if not available, chamomile roman, chamomile german, tea tree)	N, G, DS
BURSITIS:	clary sage, *cypress, juniper,* ginger, marjoram, rosemary	M, R, C
CANDIDIASIS: general	manuka, *melissa, tea tree*	SB, M, B, R
mouth	*manuka, melissa,* tea tree	MW, GR
CARBUNCLE:	cypress, lavender, ormenis flower, *ravensara, thyme linalol*	CB, C
CAR SICKNESS:	ginger, peppermint	I
CATARRH:	*cedarwood,* eucalyptus radiata, *frankincense,* myrrh, peppermint, rosemary, sandalwood, tea tree	M, R, I, B
CELLULITE:	basil, cedarwood, cypress, *fennel, juniper,* lemongrass, litsea cubeba, grapefruit, lemon, pine, rosemary	M, R, B
CHICKEN POX:	bergamot, *chamomile roman,* chamomile german, eucalyptus radiata, *lavender,* litsea cubeba, *ravensara,* tea tree	A, W, C G, S
CHILBLAINS:	chamomile german, chamomile roman, cypress, eucalyptus globulus, eucalyptus radiata, *geranium,* juniper, lavender, *lemon,* marjoram, rosemary	N, CB, C, G, R
circulation	*black pepper, geranium,* ginger, rose maroc, rosemary	N, CB, C, G, R
soothing	*chamomile roman,* marjoram, ormenis flower, sandalwood, *yuzu*	N, CB, C, G, R
itching & burning	black pepper, *chamomile german, lavender,* helichrysum, marjoram	N, CB, C, G, R

CONDITION	ESSENTIAL OILS	METHODS
swollen	*juniper, lavender,* litsea cubeba, helichrysum, marjoram	N, CB, C, G, R
CHILLS:	black pepper, *ginger,* cinnamon, clove, geranium, ormenis flower	M, R
CHILLINESS:	*black pepper, ginger,* cinnamon, clove, frankincense, marjoram	M, R
with cold hands & feet	black pepper, *geranium, ginger,* helichrysum, rosemary	M, R, B, FB,
CHILDREN: general	*lavender, chamomile roman,* mandarin, tea tree	M, R, B
sleeplessness/ worry	*lavender, chamomile roman,* mandarin	M, R, B, RF,
minor infections	*lavender, tea tree*	B, M, R, W, C, G, DR
CIRCULA-TION: poor	bay, benzoin, black pepper, cypress, frankincense, *geranium,* helichrysum, marjoram, peppermint, rose otto, rose maroc, *rosemary,* thyme linalol	M, R, B
CIRCULATORY DISORDERS:	*geranium,* helichrysum, rose maroc, *rose otto,* rosemary, vetiver	M, R, B
COLD SORES:	eucalyptus citriodora, *geranium,* manuka, *melissa, ravensara,* tea tree, yuzu	N, CB
COLDS: general	*bay,* basil, benzoin, bay, black pepper, clove, eucalyptus globulus, eucalyptus radiata, frankincense, ginger, lemon, manuka, marjoram, myrrh, orange, oregano, pine, ravensara, rosemary, tea tree, *thyme linalol*	I, M, R, B
shivering	*basil,* cinnamon, *bay,* clove, ginger, marjoram, thyme (red or linalol)	I, RF
flu-like	orange, *oregano,* ravensara, *thyme (red or linalol)*	I, RF
frequent sneezing	bay, cinnamon, *clove,* eucalyptus globulus, oregano, *pine,* thyme (red or linalol)	I, RF
runny nose	basil, *bay,* ginger	I, RF
COLITIS:	*patchouli, peppermint,* rosemary	M, R

CONDITION	ESSENTIAL OILS	METHODS
CONSTI-PATION:	black pepper, cardamom, *fennel*, mandarin, marjoram, orange, peppermint, *patchouli*, rosemary, yuzu	M, R, B
CONVALES-CENCE:	bergamot, litsea-cubeba, *mandarin*, neroli, palma rosa, petitgrain, orange, rosemary, *yuzu*	M, R, B RF
CORNS:	*lemon, tagetes,* peppermint	N, CB, FB
COUGHS: general	*benzoin*, black pepper, cardamom, cedarwood, cypress, eucalyptus globulus, eucalyptus radiata, fennel, *frankincense*, helichrysum, lemon, marjoram, myrrh, peppermint, pine, rosemary, sandalwood, tagetes, thyme linalol	R, I, RF,
dry	*cypress*, marjoram, myrrh, *sandalwood*	R, I, RF
spasmodic	*frankincense*, helichrysum, *marjoram*	R, I, RF
w/ voice-loss	frankincense, *lemon*, sandalwood, ravensara	R, I, RF
smoker's	eucalyptus globulus, *pine*, ravensara	R, I, RF
CRAMPS: general spasm	*clary sage*, cypress, *geranium*, juniper	M, R, B
after exercise	*geranium*, marjoram, rosemary,	M, R, B
recurring	*geranium, juniper,* rosemary	M, R, B
CUTS:	*lavender, tea tree*	N, G, DS
CYSTITIS: general	bergamot, chamomile roman, cedarwood, cypress, frankincense, *juniper, sandalwood,* tea tree	M, R, B, SB
pain on passing urine	*bergamot*, juniper, *sandalwood*	SB, R, B
with a temperature	*eucalyptus radiata*, chamomile roman, lavender, *sandalwood*	SB, R, B,
CYSTS:	*ormenis flower*, thyme linalol, litsea cubeba, *yuzu*	N, CB, R, C
DANDRUFF: general	cedarwood, lavender, *manuka*, patchouli, rosemary, *tea tree*	ST, W, M
w/ oily scalp	cypress, *tea tree*	ST, W, M
w/ dry scalp	rosemary, *manuka*	ST, W, M

CONDITION	ESSENTIAL OILS	METHODS
DERMATITIS:	chamomile german, geranium, *lavender,* manuka, patchouli, tea tree	M, R
DEBILITY:	*ginger,* marjoram, *petitgrain,* pine, rose otto, rosemary, thyme linalol, ylang ylang	M, R, B, RF
DENTAL INFECTIONS:	bay, *clove, myrrh,* tea tree	MW
DEPRESSION:	see following list of "Emotional States"	
DETOXIF-ICATION:	cedarwood, grapefruit, *juniper,* lemon, litsea cubeba, marjoram, orange, rosemary, vetiver, *yuzu*	B, R, M
DIARRHEA:	*black pepper, bay,* chamomile roman, clove, cinnamon, cypress, eucalyptus citriodora, ginger, peppermint, marjoram, ravensara, rosemary, sandalwood	M, R
DIGESTIVE PROBLEMS:	black pepper, coriander, *fennel,* ginger, lemon, lemongrass, mandarin, *peppermint*	M, R
DIURETIC:	black pepper, cypress, *fennel,* juniper, lemongrass, orange, sandalwood	M, R, B
DIZZINESS:	*basil,* clove, chamomile roman, *lavender*	I, RF
DROWSINESS:	*basil,* eucalyptus globulus, pine, *rosemary*	I, R
EARACHE: (otitis)	chamomile german, *lavender*	C, M, R
ECZEMA: general	benzoin, bergamot, chamomile german, *chamomile roman,* geranium, juniper, *lavender,* palmarosa, sandalwood	A, C, R, B, G, C
skin cracked & weeping	*bergamot,* frankincense, *lavender*	A, DS, C, G
sensitive to the touch	*chamomile roman, geranium,* lavender	A, R, G, C
nervous	bergamot, *lavender*	A, R, B, G, C
itching	chamomile german, *lavender, sandalwood*	R, B, G, C

CONDITION	ESSENTIAL OILS	METHODS
burning & hot	bergamot, *chamomile german, lavender*	A, R, B, G, C
ENERGY: lack of	basil, *grapefruit,* lemon, orange, rosemary	B, M, R, RF
EXHAUSTION: physical	black pepper, cardamom, clary sage, frankincense, *grapefruit,* lemon, marjoram, orange, mandarin, *palmarosa,* petitgrain, rosemary spikenard, thyme, vetiver, ylang ylang (also see following list of "Emotional States")	B, M, RF, R
FAINTING:	*basil, lavender,* peppermint, rosemary	I, RF
FATIGUE:	*basil,* bay, coriander, eucalyptus citriodora, geranium, lavender, lemon, litsea cubeba, marjoram, *pine,* palmarosa, peppermint, rosemary	B, M, RF, R
FEET: sweaty	cypress, *clary sage,* eucalyptus globulus, eucalyptus radiata, eucalyptus citriodora, geranium, peppermint, *tea tree*	B, FB, M, R
deodorants for	*clary sage,* juniper, *lemon*	FB, M, R
tired	eucalyptus citriodora, *rosemary, peppermint*	FB, M, R
FEVER:	bergamot, black pepper, chamomile german, chamomile roman, eucalyptus globulus, *eucalyptus radiata,* ginger, lemon, melissa, *ravensara,* tea tree	C, I, RF, R
FLATULENCE:	*fennel,* cardamom, coriander, *peppermint*	M, R
FLUID RETENTION:	see "Diuretic"	
FRACTURES, BONE:	*ginger*	
FRIGIDITY: (female)	clary sage, carnation, *jasmine,* rose otto, rose maroc, sandal- wood *ylang ylang*	B, M, R, RF
FUNGAL INFECTION:	see "Anti-fungal Essential Oils" list in Chapter 8	
GANGRENE:	*cinnamon,* eucalyptus globulus,	A, C, G,

CONDITION	ESSENTIAL OILS	METHODS
	lavender, *thyme linalol*, yuzu	DS, HDIL (do not massage or rub into skin, just apply on surface gently)
GASTRITIS:	lavender, *peppermint*, tea tree	R, M, B
GOUT:	*juniper*, *geranium*, helichrysum, peppermint, thyme linalol	M, R, FB, B.
GRAZES: (abrasions)	bergamot, chamomile german, *lavender*, manuka, *tea tree*	W, S, N, G, DS
GUM INFECTIONS:	manuka, *myrrh*, peppermint, thyme, *tea tree*	MW, G, R
HANGOVER:	cypress, fennel, grapefruit, *juniper*, pine, rose otto, rose maroc, *rosemary*	I, B, M, R
HAY FEVER:	*eucalyptus citriodora,* chamomile german, lavender, juniper, melissa, rose otto	I, M, B, RF
HEADACHE: general	*basil*, eucalyptus globulus, eucalyptus radiata, grapefruit, lavender, marjoram, melissa, *peppermint*, rose otto, rosemary	I, M, R, RF, B
congestive	*eucalyptus radiata*, lavender, marjoram, *peppermint*	I, M, R, RF, B
tension	chamomile roman, lavender, marjoram	I, M, R, RF, B
from travel	eucalyptus radiata, *peppermint*	I, M, R, RF, B
with a cold	eucalyptus globulus, *clove*, marjoram, *peppermint*	I, M, R, RF, B
from sinus congestion	*basil, peppermint,* eucalyptus globulus	I, M, R, RF, B
with sinusitis	*basil*, cardamom, e*ucalyptus radiata*	I, M, R, RF, B
HEARTBURN:	chamomile german, *litsea cubeba*, marjoram, *peppermint*	M, R
HEMOR-RHOIDS:	frankincense, *cypress, geranium,* marjoram, rosemary, rose maroc	A, R, B, CB, SB, LC
HERPES SIMPLEX:	bergamot, geranium, melissa	A, N, B, CB

CONDITION	ESSENTIAL OILS	METHODS
HERPES ZOSTER (shingles):	bergamot, eucalyptus radiata, geranium, *lavender*, *melissa*, ravensara	A, N, B, CB
IMMUNE STIMULANT (possible):	geranium, lavender, manuka, oregano, rosemary, thyme, yuzu	B, M, R, I, RF
immune deficiency w/ recurrent infections	geranium, lemon, manuka, melissa, rosemary, rose otto, ravensara, tea tree	B, M, R I, RF
IMPETIGO:	lavender, *manuka*, tea tree, *thyme linalol*, ravensara	B, R
IMPOTENCE: (male)	clary sage, *cardamom*, *ginger*, ormenis flower, sandalwood, *vetiver*, ylang ylang	M, B, R, RF
INDIGESTION:	*cardamom*, *fennel*, coriander, ginger, lemon, peppermint	M, R, C
INFECTIONS: general	bergamot, black pepper, cinnamon, juniper, lavender, lemon, lemongrass, manuka, myrrh, oregano, pine, ravensara, rosemary, tea tree, thyme (linalol or red), yuzu (Most essential oils help to fight infection to some degree. See also "Anti-Infectious Essential Oils" list in Chapter 8)	A, M, R, C, B, G, W, DS
INFLUENZA (flu):	*bay*, black pepper, *cinnamon*, clove, cypress, eucalyptus radiata, eucalyptus globulus, basil, ginger, lemon, manuka, ravensara, peppermint, oregano, thyme linalol	M, RF, I
INFLAM-MATION:	*chamomile german,* chamomile roman, *lavender*	A, B, R C, G, DS
INSECT REPELLENT:	*cedarwood, citronella,* eucalyptus citriodora, *lavender,* patchouli, peppermint, sandalwood	RF
INSOMNIA: general	chamomile roman, *lavender*, linden blossom, clary sage, neroli, marjoram, *ormenis flower*, petitgrain, sandalwood, ylang ylang	B, M, R, RF
restlessness	lavender, *chamomile roman*, neroli	B, M, R, RF

CONDITION	ESSENTIAL OILS	METHODS
over-tired	*clary sage*, lavender, *ormenis flower*	B, M, R, RF
nightmares	chamomile roman, *frankincense, lavender*	B, M, R, RF
worry	clary sage, *ormenis flower,* ylang ylang, *yuzu*	B, M, R, RF
depression	lavender, *neroli*, sandalwood, *ylang ylang*	B, M, R, RF
physical causes	chamomile roman, *lavender, marjoram*	B, M, R, RF
JET LAG:	*basil*, geranium, *grapefruit, juniper*, peppermint, rosemary	B, M, R, I, RF
JOINTS: swollen	helichrysum, *litsea cubeba*, chamomile roman, *juniper*, rosemary, lavender, fennel (see "Arthritis" and "Rheumatism")	B, M, R, C
painful	*basil, black pepper*, cedarwood, chamomile, *ginger*, helichrysum, lavender, rosemary, thyme (red or linalol)	B, M, R, C
strained	bay, *black pepper, cedarwood,* clary sage, *ginger,* helichrysum, lavender, rosemary	B, M, R, C
LARYNGITIS: general	*benzoin*, bergamot, cypress, geranium, lavender, *lemon, thyme linalol*	G, MW
loss of voice	*geranium*, grapefruit, *lemon*	G, MW
tickling throat	*benzoin*, clove, grapefruit, *lemon*	G, MW
LICE: body	lavender, *manuka, tea tree*	B, M, R, W, N
head	lavender, *manuka, tea tree*	B, M, R, W
LIGAMENTS: painful from over-exertion	black pepper, *lemongrass, rosemary*	M, R, C
LIVER PROBLEMS:	chamomile roman, cypress, *fennel*, geranium, grapefruit, juniper, *lemon*, mandarin, peppermint, rosemary, thyme linalol	C, B, M, R
LYMPHATIC CONGESTION:	fennel, *geranium*, juniper, lavender, manuka, ravensara, *yuzu*	M, R, B
MEASLES:	*bergamot, chamomile german*, eucalyptus citriodora, eucalyptus	A, C, B, R, I

CONDITION	ESSENTIAL OILS	METHODS
	radiata, geranium, lavender, manuka, *ravensara*, tea tree, thyme	
MEMORY ENHANCE- MENT:	*rosemary, basil*	I, RF
MENOPAUSE: general	chamomile roman, *clary sage*, cypress, *geranium*, jasmine, lavender, neroli, *rose maroc*, sandalwood	B, M, R, RF
depression	bergamot, benzoin, *geranium*, neroli, *rose otto*	B, M, R, RF
insomnia	chamomile roman, clary sage, marjoram, *spikenard, vetiver*	B, M, R, RF
hot flashes	chamomile roman, *clary sage*, eucalyptus radiata, fennel, geranium, lavender, *yuzu*	B (cool), M, R, S
perspiration, excessive	clary sage, *cypress*	B (cool), R, S
MENSTRUAL PROBLEMS:	(for premenstral syndrome see "PMS")	
amenorrhea (absence of periods)	*clary sage*, fennel, *geranium*, rose maroc	M, R, B
irregular/ scanty periods	*clary sage*, fennel, geranium, *rose maroc*	M, R, B
dysmenor- rhea (painful periods)	bay, *clary sage,* chamomile roman, clove, *geranium*, helichrysum, lavender, marjoram, peppermint, rose maroc	M, R, B, SB
menorrhagia (excessive bleeding)	cypress, *frankincense*, geranium, jasmine, rose maroc	M, R, B
breast tenderness	*chamomile roman,* lavender, geranium, *marjoram*	C, M, R, B
MIGRAINE: general	chamomile roman, lavender, marjoram, *peppermint, rosemary*	C, R, N
allergy	lavender, *juniper,* rose otto, *yuzu*	B, M
tension	chamomile roman, *lavender, peppermint*, yuzu	B, M

CONDITION	ESSENTIAL OILS	METHODS
MOUTH INFECTIONS:	geranium, manuka, *myrrh*, *tea tree*	MW, M (outer jaw)
MOUTH ULCERS:	lemon, manuka, *myrrh, tea tree*	CB
MUCOUS CONGESTION:	eucalyptus radiata, *eucalyptus globulas*, eucalyptus citriodora, frankincense, peppermint, *ravensara*, rosemary, thyme linalol	M, R, B, I, RF
MUMPS:	*chamomile german, lavender,* helichrysum, *litsea cubeba*, manuka, tea tree, thyme linalol	M, R, C
MUSCULAR: aches	basil, bay, black pepper, chamomile roman, *clary sage*, eucalyptus globulus, ginger, helichrysum, *marjoram, ormenis flower*, peppermint, rosemary, thyme linalol, vetiver	M, R, B
cramps	cardamom, clary sage, geranium, ginger, *helichrysum*, peppermint, *rosemary*	M, R, B, C
debility	basil, *ginger*, juniper, lavender, *marjoram*, ormenis flower, thyme linalol	M, R, B
fatigue	bay, *black pepper*, clary sage, ginger, grapefruit, *juniper*, lavender, lemongrass, pine	M, R, B
numbness	*benzoin, black pepper*, cinnamon, clove, geranium, ginger, helichrysum, marjoram	R, M, B, C
pain	basil, bay, black pepper, clove, eucalyptus, globulus, eucalyptus radiata, ginger, *helichrysum*, marjoram, manuka, oregano, *peppermint*, pine, ravensara, rosemary, *thyme linalol*, thyme red, yuzu	M, R, B, C
relaxant	benzoin, chamomile roman, *clary sage*, lavender, marjoram, ormenis flower, *spikenard, vetiver*, ylang ylang	M, R, B
spasm	basil, bergamot, cardamom, chamomile roman, *clary sage*, clove, coriander, cypress, fennel,	M, R, B, C

CONDITION	ESSENTIAL OILS	METHODS
	geranium, helichrysum, jasmine, lavender, marjoram, ormenis flower, *peppermint*, petitgrain, *rosemary*, thyme linalol, vetiver	
NAIL FUNGUS:	*tea tree*, tagetes, melissa, *manuka*	R, CB
NAUSEA: general	clove, fennel, *ginger*, melissa, *peppermint*, sandalwood	I, RF, M, R
migraine-induced	lavender, *peppermint*	I, M, R, RF
from over-eating	coriander, *fennel*	I, M, R, RF
from traveling	*ginger*, peppermint	I, M, R, RF
NECK, STIFF:	*basil,* clary sage, ginger, lavender, peppermint, *rosemary*	B, M, R
NETTLE RASH:	*chamomile german*, *chamomile roman*, *lavender*, tea tree, yuzu	N, R
NEURALGIA:	*bay*, benzoin, *black pepper*, chamomile roman, *chamomile german*, clary sage, eucalyptus radiata, *geranium*, marjoram, peppermint, yuzu	B, M, R, C
NOSE BLEED:	cypress, frankincense, lavender, lemon	C
OBESITY:	eucalyptus radiata, *fennel, juniper*, lemon, litsea cubeba, oregano, ravensara, rosemary, thyme, yuzu	B, M, R
OVERINDUL- GENCE: general	juniper, *grapefruit, lemon*, orange, rosemary, vetiver	I, RF, R B, C
alcohol	*fennel*, grapefruit, *juniper*, lemon, peppermint, *rosemary*, yuzu	I, R, M, B, C
OVERWEIGHT:	fennel, *grapefruit*, juniper, lemon, patchouli, petitgrain, *yuzu*	B, M, R
OVER-WORK:	*clary sage*, jasmine, lavender, *litsea cubeba*, neroli, rosemary, ylang ylang, yuzu	B, M, R, RF
PARASITIC INFESTATION:	lavender, *manuka, patchouli*, peppermint, tagetes, tea tree	A, R, B, W, HDIL
PMS:	*clary sage*, chamomile roman, fennel,	B, M,

CONDITION	ESSENTIAL OILS	METHODS
general	*geranium*, neroli, rosemary, ylang ylang	R
depression	*bergamot*, chamomile roman, *geranium*, rose otto	B, M, R
irritability	bergamot, chamomile roman, *geranium*, lavender, *yuzu*	B, M, R
moodiness	*bergamot*, *geranium*, grapefruit, lavender, mandarin	B, M, R
tender breasts	*chamomile roman*, chamomile german, geranium, *lavender*, marjoram	B, M, R
water retention (bloating)	cypress, *fennel*, *juniper* (see also "Diuretic")	B, M, R
weepiness	*benzoin*, geranium, neroli, *rose otto*	B, M, R

PREGNANCY:

pre-natal (third trimester)	jasmine, *rose otto*, *sandalwood*, ylang ylang	B, M, R, RF
birth	*jasmine, rose otto*, yuzu	B, M, R, RF
morning sickness	cardamom, *coriander*, *ginger*, peppermint	I, R, RF
post-natal	*bergamot*, lavender, frankincense, *neroli*	B, M, R, RF
refreshing (all times)	geranium, *grapefruit*, *lavender*, litsea cubeba, rose otto, *yuzu*	R, M, B
breast feeding	*fennel, geranium*	R, M, B
post-natal depression	*bergamot*, chamomile roman, geranium, jasmine, *neroli*, rose otto, *yuzu*	B, M, R, RF
sleep disturbed	chamomile roman, *lavender*	B, M, R, RF
stretch marks (third trimester)	neroli, petitgrain, geranium, jasmine	M, R

PSORIASIS:	benzoin, *bergamot*, chamomile roman, geranium, *lavender*	M, R, C, G
RASHES:	chamomile german, chamomile roman, eucalyptus globulus, eucalyptus radiata, *lavender*, tea tree	B, R, G, C, DS
RAYNARD'S DISEASE:	clove, *geranium*, marjoram, *rose maroc*	B, M, R
RESPIRATORY PROBLEMS:	basil, *benzoin*, cedarwood, eucalyptus globulus, frankincense,	B, M, R, I

CONDITION	ESSENTIAL OILS	METHODS
general	oregano, peppermint, *ravensara*, rosemary, sandalwood, thyme (red or linalol)	
infections	cinnamon, clove, oregano, *ravensara, thyme (red or linalol)*	R, I, RF
RHEUMATISM:	*bay*, benzoin, *black pepper*, cedarwood, chamomile german, chamomile roman, clove, coriander, cypress, eucalyptus citriodora, eucalyptus globulus, eucalyptus radiata, frankincense, ginger, *helichrysum*, juniper, lavender, lemon, manuka, marjoram, oregano, peppermint, pine, *rosemary*, thyme (red or linalol), vetiver	B, M, R
RINGWORM:	clove, *manuka*, myrrh, *patchouli*, tea tree	A, N, C, W, CB
SCABIES:	clove, cinnamon, lemon, *manuka*, myrrh, oregano, *tea tree*, thyme linalol	A, CB, C, W, B
SCALP DISORDERS:	cedarwood, lavender, *manuka*, rosemary, *tea tree*	R, M
SCAR TISSUE:	jasmine, *neroli*, palmarosa, petitgrain, *rosehip*, rose otto, rose maroc, sandalwood	M, R, FO
SCIATICA:	*chamomile roman*, chamomile german, *lavender*, helichrysum, juniper, peppermint	C, M, R, N
SEA-SICKNESS:	*ginger*	I
SHOCK (physical):	*basil, lavender*, peppermint (see also following list of "Emotional States")	
SINUSITIS: general	*basil*, eucalyptus globulus, eucalyptus radiata, lavender, marjoram, peppermint, *pine*, ravensara, *rosemary*, tea tree	N, M, R, I
w/ head pain	eucalyptus globulus, *peppermint*, ravensara, *rosemary* (see also "Headache")	N, M, R, I
w/ congestion	*basil*, peppermint, *rosemary*	N, M, R, I
with catarrh	*eucalyptus globulus*, eucalyptus radiata, *pine*	N, M, R, I

CONDITION	ESSENTIAL OILS	METHODS
SKIN CARE: general	chamomile german, chamomile roman, fennel, frankincense, jasmine, lavender, lemon, lemongrass, litsea cubeba, mandarin, myrrh, *neroli*, orange, palmarosa, petitgrain, *rose otto*, rose maroc, rosemary, sandalwood, ylang ylang, yuzu (also see "Acne" and "Eczema")	FO, S, FT, C, LC, FM
skin infections	bay, bergamot, *lavender*, litsea cubeba, manuka, rose otto, rose maroc, *tea tree*, ylang ylang, yuzu	FO, S, W, C
aging/mature	clary sage, frankincense, geranium, *neroli*, patchouli, *petitgrain*, *rose otto*, sandalwood	FO, S, FT, LC FM
allergies	chamomile german, *chamomile roman*, *lavender*	FO, S, FT, C
blackheads	cypress, *rosemary*, yuzu	FO, S, W, FT, FM, C, LC
blotches	geranium, *lavender*, *rose otto*, chamomile roman	FO, S, FT, C, LC
broken veins	cypress, *geranium*, neroli, *sandalwood*	FO, S, FT, C, LC
redness	chamomile roman, *chamomile german*, lavender	FO, S, FT, C, LC
burning sensation	chamomile roman, *chamomile german*, lavender	FO, S, FT, LC, C
chapped	*benzoin*, geranium, myrrh, *sandalwood*, yuzu	FO, R, LC
cracked	*benzoin*, frankincense, patchouli	FO, R, C, LC
dry	chamomile, geranium, jasmine, neroli, *rose otto*, sandalwood	FO, LC, FM
greasy (prone to infections)	bergamot, cypress, geranium, grapefruit, lavender, lemon	FO, S, W, FT, C, FM, LC
inflamed	*chamomile german*, clary sage, frankincense, geranium, *lavender*, sandalwood, tea tree	FO, S, LC, FT, C
itchy	chamomile roman, *frankincense*, lavender	FO, LC

CONDITION	ESSENTIAL OILS	METHODS
irritated	benzoin, chamomile german, *lavender*, sandalwood	FO, S, LC, C
normal	geranium, *jasmine*, *neroli*, sandalwood, ylang ylang	FO, S, FT, FM, C
oily	bergamot, cedarwood, *cypress*, *geranium*, juniper, rosemary, sandalwood, *ylang ylang*	FO, S, FM, LC, C
sensitive	*chamomile roman*, geranium, lavender, neroli, *rose otto*	FO, LC, FM
SORES:	eucalyptus citriodora, *lavender*, manuka, myrrh, *tea tree*, yuzu	A, C, CB, G, DS
STRESS:	see following list of "Emotional States"	
SUNBURN:	chamomile roman, eucalyptus radiata, *lavender*	C, B, N
THROAT: sore	eucalyptus radiata, eucalyptus citriodora, fennel, *lemon*, sandalwood	MW, R, C, G
dry	lavender, *sandalwood*	MW, R, C, G
burning	chamomile roman, eucalyptus citriodora, frankincense, *lavender*, *lemon*	MW, R, C, G
infections	geranium, *lemon*, manuka, sandalwood, *tea tree*, thyme linalol	MW, R, C, G
irritated	cypress, *frankincense*, geranium, lemon	MW, R, C, G
THRUSH	see "Candidiasis"	
TIREDNESS: mental	*basil*, grapefruit, lemon, *peppermint*, *rosemary*, yuzu	I, RF, B, M
physical	basil, bay, clary sage, *grapefruit*, lavender, marjoram, *rosemary*	M, R, B
TONIC, GENERAL:	cedarwood, chamomile roman, *eucalyptus citriodora*, frankincense, helichrysum, lemon, lemongrass, *litsea cubeba*, melissa, *orange*, ravensara, rose maroc, rose otto, *rosemary*, yuzu	M, R, B
TONSILLITIS:	chamomile roman, *lavender*, manuka, *tea tree*, yuzu, thyme linalol	MW, G, R

CONDITION	ESSENTIAL OILS	METHODS
TOOTHACHE:	chamomile roman, *clove*, peppermint	C, MW, CB, M (outer jaw)
TRAUMA:	*benzoin*, bergamot, chamomile roman, *lavender*, linden blossom, *rose otto*, rose maroc, yuzu (see also following lists of "Emotional States")	B, M, R, I, RF
ULCERATIONS:	benzoin, chamomile german, eucalyptus globulus, eucalyptus radiata, geranium, juniper, *lavender*, myrrh, tea tree	A, C, G DS, W, S, CB
VARICOSE VEINS:	*cypress, geranium*, juniper, lemon	A, B, R, C
VERUCCAS: (plantar warts)	clove, *lemon*, manuka, oregano, tea tree, *thyme (red)*	A, C, W, CB, FB
VIRAL INFECTIONS:	see "Anti-Viral Essential Oils" list in Chapter 8	
post-viral conditions	eucalyptus citriodora, fennel, frankincense, *geranium,* grapefruit, *juniper, lemon*, tea tree, yuzu	B, M, R, I, F
WARTS:	clove, *lemon*, manuka, oregano, tea tree, *thyme (red or linalol)*	A, N, C, CB
WHITLOW: (inflammation with pus on finger or toe)	bergamot, *chamomile roman*, *lavender*, tea tree, thyme	A, N C, CB
WINDBURN:	chamomile german, chamomile roman, lavender	FO, S
WOUNDS:	benzoin, bergamot, chamomile roman, eucalyptus citriodora, frankincense, *lavender*, manuka, myrrh, *tea tree*	W, N, C, S

EMOTIONAL STATE	ESSENTIAL OILS	METHODS
ANXIETY:	*benzoin*, bergamot, cedarwood, *chamomile roman*, *clary sage*, eucalyptus citriodora, jasmine, lavender, linden blossom, litsea cubeba, marjoram, *neroli*, patchouli, petitgrain, rose maroc, sandalwood, spikenard, ylang ylang, yuzu	B, I, M, R, RF
CALMING:	bay, benzoin, bergamot, carnation, chamomile roman, clary sage, eucalyptus citriodora, *hyacinth*, *lavender*, linden blossom, mandarin, marjoram, melissa, neroli, *ormenis flower*, petitgrain, rose maroc, rose otto, sandalwood, vetiver, ylang ylang, yuzu	B, I, M, R, RF
CONCENTRATION: (lack of)	*basil*, black pepper, *cardamom*, ginger	B, I, M, R, RF
DEPRESSION:	*benzoin*, *bergamot*, carnation, chamomile roman, clary sage, frankincense, geranium, grapefruit, *jasmine*, lavender, lemon, linden blossom, *litsea cubeba*, melissa, *neroli*, ormenis flower, patchouli, petitgrain, rose maroc, *rose otto*, sandalwood, *ylang ylang*, yuzu	B, I, M, R, RF
EMOTIONAL CRISIS:	*benzoin*, bergamot, hyacinth, *linden blossom*, *rose otto*, rose maroc	B, I, M, R, RF
FEAR:	bergamot, chamomile roman, *frankincense*, ginger, *lavender*, neroli, spikenard, *vetiver*	B, I, M, R, RF
HYSTERIA:	bergamot, chamomile roman, *lavender*, linden blossom, melissa, *spikenard*	B, I, M, R, RF
IRRITABILITY:	benzoin, *chamomile roman*, clary sage, geranium, lavender, neroli, mandarin, marjoram, *ormenis flower*, petitgrain, sandalwood, vetiver, ylang ylang	B, I, M, R, RF

EMOTIONAL STATE	ESSENTIAL OILS	METHODS
MENTAL EXHAUSTION:	*basil*, eucalyptus citriodora, eucalyptus globulus, eucalyptus radiata, grapefruit, juniper, lemon, *pine*, yuzu	B, I, M, R, RF
MENTAL TIREDNESS:	basil, cardamom, coriander, frankincense, *grapefruit*, hyacinth, *rosemary*, peppermint	B, I, M, R, RF
NERVOUS-NESS:	chamomile roman, clary sage, cypress, geranium, jasmine, *lavender*, lemongrass, litsea cubeba, neroli, ormenis flower, palmarosa, *vetiver*, *ylang ylang*	B, I, M, R RF
NERVOUS TENSION:	benzoin, clary sage, jasmine, juniper, *lavender*, linden blossom, mandarin, marjoram, ormenis flower, palmarosa, rose otto, rose maroc, *sandalwood*, spikenard, vetiver, ylang ylang, yuzu	B, I, M, R, RF
RELAXING:	benzoin, bergamot, carnation, chamomile roman, clary sage, eucalyptus citriodora, geranium, hyacinth, jasmine, lavender, linden blossom, litsea cubeba, neroli, ormenis flower, palmarosa, petitgrain, rose otto, rose maroc, sandalwood, vetiver, ylang ylang	B, I, M, R, RF
SHOCK (emotional):	benzoin, *lavender*, neroli, rose otto	B, I, M, R, RF
SORROW:	*benzoin*, hyacinth, linden blossom, *rose otto*	B, I, M, R, RF
STRESS:	basil, benzoin, bergamot, carnation, *chamomile roman*, clary sage, clove, frankincense, *geranium*, hyacinth, *jasmine*, lavender, lemon, linden blossom, litsea cubeba, mandarin, marjoram, melissa, *neroli, ormenis flower*, palmarosa, patchouli, petitgrain, *rose maroc*, rose otto, sandalwood, vetiver, *ylang ylang*, yuzu	B, I, R, M, RF
TENSION:	bergamot, chamomile roman,	B, I, M,

EMOTIONAL STATE	ESSENTIAL OILS	METHODS
	cypress, frankincense, *geranium*, hyacinth, jasmine, *lavender*, mandarin, marjoram, neroli, ormenis flower, petitgrain, rose maroc, sandalwood, *spikenard*, *vetiver*, ylang ylang	R, RF

Chapter 7

Good Health

Diet and Herbal Teas

The most important thing to remember about diet is this: include enough fresh food so that your body gets the vitamins and minerals it needs. The *problem* with this "good advice" is that today's vegetables, fruits, and grains are subjected to so many processes in production — including pesticide, fungicide, and herbicide treatment, waxing, and irradiation — that the fresh purity has been processed out of our food. We can remedy this by using as much organic produce as possible and by taking supplements of natural vitamins, minerals, nutrients, and enzymes.

Vitamins, the vital building blocks of

life, are found in great quantities in foods but are also found in small amounts in herbal teas, and in minute quantities in some essential oils. For example, there is vitamin C in lemon essential oil. Some essential oils also contain tiny quantities of minerals, drawn by the plant from the earth.

We employ a form of aromatic medicine when we use herbs in our cooking. Whereas in times past the herbs would have been plucked fresh and organic from the garden, now they are more likely to be commercially grown. chemically sprayed and then dried, irradiated, and packaged. Mildew could easily form if the producers washed the herbs, so they avoid it. For this reason, when buying herbs, try to ensure they come from health food shops and other suppliers of organic produce. Alternatively, try growing a few pots in your garden or window box. The seeds are usually easy to obtain and by growing your own you can be sure of a fresh supply. Herbs can be used to make herb teas as well as in cooking.

To make an herb tea, cut up about a teaspoon of herb (per cup), put it in the cup and pour boiling water on it, then place a saucer over the top to prevent the steam from escaping. Let it cool down, then strain and drink. All over the world many people use mint tea to help alleviate intestinal discomfort or flatulence, or just to enjoy the taste, but any kind of herb that you can use in cooking can also be used to make a tea. Choices might include basil, marjoram, thyme, chamomile, melissa, and spearmint — these last two make a good blend. Even lavender flowers can be made into a tea. A beautiful red color is produced in tea made with hibiscus flowers, which is said to be full of vitamin C. If you are lucky enough to have an orange or lemon tree growing in your garden (and can be sure no biocide residues or wax are on the peel) dry the peel of the fruit, grate it, and put it in teas. With all the possible options, there are many combinations of teas to try.

If you grow your own herbs, wash them before drying. To avoid mildew forming, dry them as quickly as possible hanging upside down, in a place with warm, circulating air. Many varieties of herbs can also be bought from specialty shops. These also sell kits for making tea bags and it can be great fun, and convenient, to make up your own personalized mixes of teas for future use.

Herbs can also be used in salads and sauces. If you have a favorite sauce recipe, you can enhance its taste to make it even more nutritious by adding lots of fresh herbs. In Switzerland, the locals make a "green sauce" from chopped herbs which is especially relished poured over boiled potatoes. Flavored salad and cooking oils can be made by adding fresh herbs to olive oil, and/or adding a couple of drops of the same essential oil to each pint of olive oil.

Another way to add purity and health to your life is to diffuse essential oils in the atmosphere, to bathe daily with essential oils, and to use essential oil "massage oils" — which can simply be applied to the skin like a body oil, as well as used as a massage treatment.

Exercise

Although we are constantly told that exercise is good for us, how many of us do it regularly? People say "it's boring," but the answer is to find a form of it that suits you. If two minutes of stretching each morning is as much as you can handle, fine, but first use a body-scrubber, a loofa, or plastic glove, stroking the skin towards the heart, to get the blood circulating. One minute of body scrubbing and two minutes of stretching really sets you up for a good day.

While going about your everyday business, try to speed up and get the muscles working. Your metabolism can be increased simply by walking that little bit faster and not dawdling, and sprinting up the stairs instead of walking. Every daily activity can be turned into an exercise. As you walk through long corridors, concentrate on the action of the leg muscles, making them work. If commuting by bus or train, do stomach contractions as you read the daily paper. A toe-touching workout can be done during a quiet moment — just let the head fall forward, bending your body from the hips. Relax deeply and the weight of your head will slowly pull the body downward, unlocking the spine. Relax deeply. You don't actually have to touch your toes; only go as far as you can in a relaxed manner. Relaxation is the key to the success of this exercise. The back of the legs can be exercised while sitting at your desk: Push off your shoes, raise your legs slightly, then stretch and point your toes downward, then push your heels down, and so on. Now turn your ankle in small circles, one way and then the other — this helps prevent fluid accumulating in the ankle.

Even if you can only manage two or three minutes of exercise a day, that is a good thing. It helps to be regular about exercise and it is easier to keep to a regimen that is workable — if two minutes a day is all you can manage, make it each and every day.

There are so many different sports it is difficult to imagine that there is not at least one to suit each of us. However, we may not all have easy access to the facilities, or the money to pay for equipment or transport. If that's the problem, try to borrow a bicycle, and make that your sport. Going somewhere for a picnic with a friend on a bicycle is a joy as well as exercise. People take great pleasure from sports and they are not all expensive, but if "sport for sport's sake" doesn't appeal to you, think of a sport that has some other purpose — such as self-defense.

It is difficult to find time to exercise when you work all day and then have to shop for dinner and cook, and all the rest. But even one stretch is better than nothing and five stretches are better than that. Don't be unrealistic in your demands upon yourself. Decide what you can easily do and later, if you wish, gradually expand on the time spent doing it. Exercise doesn't have to be punishment, and it is so very good for us — keeping us fit, supple, and younger. Lack of muscle tone in the face can make a face "drop," so exercise here is important, too. Open the mouth as far as you can, grimace, and open eyes as wide as you can. Relax and repeat three times. Remember that whatever blood goes around the body also circulates around the brain; good circulation helps you think.

Exercise stimulates good metabolism, circulation, muscle tone, health, and beauty. The crucial thing is not to overdo it — making things worse than they were to begin with. Watch out for straining muscles and be careful lifting and making other movements. Push yourself by all means, but in small incremental steps, using common sense.

*P*ositive Thinking

We all employ positive thinking to different degrees. You had a positive thought when you purchased this book — taking responsibility for your health. If it was a gift to you, someone else had the positive thought. People differ in their relative negative-positive approach to life. Some see the bottle as half-full, and others see it as half-empty. But, as research increasingly shows, positive thinking can lead to positive health. The mind-body connection is now an accepted scientific fact.[6]

Thinking positively doesn't mean building castles in the air — dreaming dreams that will never be realized, or at least not this week. You can't become a ballet dancer if you haven't taken any dance lessons! Think within the scope of possibility; be realistic. That way, you won't leave yourself open to disappointment. Lay plans — bricks on the path leading inexorably forward — but lay one at a time; don't set yourself too many tasks. Be positive about what you know and can

---

[6]See *The Fragrant Mind* by Valerie Ann Worwood, London: Doubleday, 1995.

realistically do, aiming to build on your knowledge and experience.

Many people find positive affirmations very helpful. The idea is to repeat your personal affirmation regularly. You might say or think "I am special," and repeat that over and over. Do it as you dress, or sit on the train going to work. Or your affirmation might be "I can do this job." As you say it to yourself over and over, regularly each day, the thought becomes a nugget of truth deep within you which can be latched onto for strength and support during difficult moments. A good time to do positive affirmation is while massaging yourself with essential oils.

Self Massage

Although aromatherapy uses the term "massage oil" to describe a dilution of essential oils in base, vegetable, or carrier oil, these "massage oils" can be used the same way as one would use any body oil or lotion — simply applied, rubbed on, or smoothed onto the skin. This certainly allows us to absorb the benefits of the essential oils and their therapeutic properties. However, the benefit of diluted essential oils is increased if they can be applied during the process of massage. In an ideal world, we would all have access to a daily aromatherapy massage at home, but the reality is that we do not always have a person who can do the massage for us. This need not be a problem because it is not difficult to massage oneself.

The following routine can, with practice, be done in about ten minutes. I have given guidelines to repeat each part three times but you may feel the need to spend more time on particular areas. Also, portions of the massage can be done on their own. Enjoy taking this time to pamper yourself. You deserve it, and the aromatherapy self-massage is about promoting health. It just happens to be a great pleasure and so feels like an indulgence!

Prepare a massage oil using your chosen essential oils. You will need no more than approximately 15 mls or 3 teaspoons (½ oz) of oil. This massage is very effective after a shower or bath as the body's dead skin cells have been washed away and the body will be warm. Do the massage in a comfortable room where you will not be disturbed. Protect any bedclothes or furnishing material by sitting on a large towel — one you can wrap yourself into after you have finished the massage.

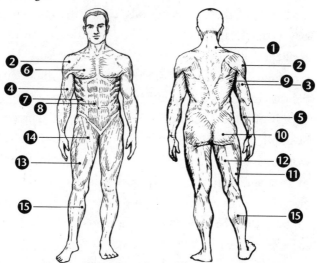

Refer to these drawings of the human muscle structure
to locate the muscles discussed in this section.

Start by pouring a little massage oil into your hand and smooth it all over your chest, shoulders, and arms.

Shoulders

The following massage movements will release the tension that gathers in the shoulder muscles, improve posture, and stimulate circulation in the neck and face.

Trapezius Muscle ❶

• Using your right hand, grasp your left shoulder muscle firmly, gathering as much flesh or muscle as you can between your palm and fingers, and slowly squeeze, then release, the muscle.

• Slide your fingers from your neck outwards towards the shoulder, using small circular massage movements until you reach the top of the arm. Repeat this as often as you like.

Deltoid Muscle ❷

• Now keep the right hand in a relaxed position, and with the whole hand massage your shoulder in one large circular movement which should be in an outwards direction — down over the back of the shoulder and up across the front.

• Massaging with all your fingers, slide down the top and back of the shoulder, and repeat.

• Using a soothing but firm movement, sweep down the whole arm, up around the shoulder, and up around the back of the neck.

• Repeat the whole movement three times.

• Now use the left hand and repeat all the movements on the right side.

Arms

Arm massage improves skin tone and texture and increases circulation. It can be done at any time to ease aches and pains. The arm massage is followed by the hand massage, in sequence. Start with one arm and continue on to the hand, then massage your other arm and hand in the same way.

Triceps ❸ *and Biceps Muscles* ❹

• Rest your hand on your lap. Grip as much of your upper arm as you can and, using circular movements, massage your upper arm firmly. Much of this will entail lifting the muscles and flesh.

• Now, using the whole palm and all the fingers, tap firmly but gently all over the upper arm. This increases circulation and helps gets rid of small bumps under the skin that can gather on the arm.

Flexors/Extensors Muscles ❺

• Using the heel of your hand and fingers, and using small round movements, massage your forearm.

• Massage around the elbow then slowly slide your hand down until you reach your other hand and repeat the tapping movements on the whole forearm area.

• Continue on to the hand massage.

Hands

The hand massage will keep your hands and fingers supple and improve skin tone. It is especially valuable for people who use their hands a lot, like keyboard operators and musicians — and helps keep complaints such as rheumatism at bay — although everyone can benefit. Do the movements as many times you wish.

• With your hand still resting on your lap, turn the palm upward, supporting that hand with the fingers and palm of the massaging hand. Massage the palm of the hand with the thumb.

• Holding each finger in turn between your forefinger and thumb, massage each finger with gentle rolling movements, as if rolling a marble between your thumb and forefinger. Pay particular attention to the joints. Always starting at the tips, massage up the finger exerting pressure to upper and lower surfaces; then massage up the finger concentrating on the sides, between the fingers.

• Keep your hand relaxed and resting on your knee but turn it over and massage each knuckle separately.

• Lay the palm of your hand down on your thigh and with your thumb gently glide up between the tendons of each finger, on the back of the hand.

• Using the palm and fingers, smooth over the hand and up the whole arm using a sweeping massage movement.

• Now massage your other arm and hand using the same sequence.

Chest and Breasts

By using an aromatherapy massage oil on the chest, you can help release tension in the muscles of the neck and shoulders, lift the breast, and keep the skin toned.

Pectoralis Major 6

• Place your right hand at the center of the upper chest and slide it firmly outward toward your left shoulder, under the collarbone. Repeat the movement but this time do it directly underneath the previous one, closer to the armpit. Gradually move down the upper chest an inch at a time until you reach the top of the breast.

• Repeat on the other side using the other hand.

• Only use very gentle circular movements to massage the breasts, working around the outside of the breasts themselves. Massage both breasts at the same time, using one hand for each breast. Slide your hand down the side of the breast cupping and lifting gently, then slide your hand up the sternum. Turn the elbows out at this point and continue the movement across the top of the breast. Repeat.

Abdomen

Abdominal massage can be carried out while sitting, standing, or lying down. These movements will help increase circulation and improve the tone and texture of the skin. It also helps the movement of the intestines. This massage can be carried out separately if needed, for example if you have abdominal bloating, cramps, constipation, or other abdominal discomforts.

Obliquus Externus 7 and Rectus Abdominis 8

• Using one hand in a clockwise movement, sweep

around the whole abdomen with a smooth but firm movement.

• Continue this clockwise circular movement around the umbilicus (the navel), this time using both hands, one following the other in the direction of intestinal flow.

• Again using two hands, one following the other in the clockwise direction, take hold of the flesh and roll it between your thumbs and fingers. Cover the whole abdomen always moving in the same direction.

Hips and Back

Sacroiliac Bone and Latissimus Dorsi Muscle ❾

• Place both hands on your hips, at the back, and slowly smooth over your hip bones with a firm, smooth movement.

• Place both hands on your hips with your thumbs at the back and facing each other on either side of the vertebra. Use small circular massage movements using only your thumb, and work around the hip and the bone at the lower back. You can work quite deeply into the fleshy areas. This is a wonderful movement if you have lower back pain. Repeat as often as you like.

Latissimus Dorsi Muscle ❾

• Place both hands on your hip at the back, in the same way as before with the thumbs facing each other at either side of the vertebra. Using the same circular thumb movements work up the back as far as you can go. Repeat this movement as many times you like, finishing the sequence with your hands on your hips.

• Place both hands on your hips behind your back, with your fingers facing each other, and your thumbs resting on your hipbone at the side. Make the same circular massage movements — but this time using the fingers and palm of the hand, massage up either side of the vertebra, moving up as far as you can. Each time you do this movement you'll find you are able to travel just that little bit higher up the large latissimus muscles on either side of the vertebra.

• When you find that you can't travel up the back any farther, start moving down the back muscle again but make sure the pressure is applied on the upward sweep of the circle.

• Turning your hands, make a large, smooth, sweeping movement over the hips.

Buttocks

These movements increase circulation, remove toxins, ease tension out and improve skin tone. They are very useful for those who have to sit at work for long periods of time.

Gluteus Maximus 🔟

• Using both hands, make a large sweeping movement over the whole of each buttock going towards the sides of the body, not the center.

• With the fingertips and thumb, use small circular massage movements, gradually making the movements smaller, and quicker, and slightly deeper into the muscle each time.

• Knead the flesh and muscles of the buttocks using one hand on each buttock as if kneading dough, taking the flesh between fingers and thumb.

• Finish this section of the massage with large sweeping movements over the whole buttock and hip area.

Legs

A leg massage will increase circulation, improve muscle tone, and gradually ease out any aches and any pains. These movements are very helpful if you have over-exercised muscles. To begin, smooth some massage oil all over the leg, from top to bottom, using both hands.

Biceps Femoris ⓫ *and Semi-tendinosus* ⓬

• Start with the portion of the leg above the knee. Work upwards from the knee massaging the side and back of your leg. Use firm, kneading movements, taking the flesh and muscle between your fingers and thumbs. Gather the flesh as best you can, and knead it, while moving slowly upward toward the buttocks using one hand after the other.

Rectus Femoris ⓭

• Do the same movement, now on the top of the thigh starting at the knee.

Sartorius ⓮

• Do the same movement on the inside of the thigh starting at the knee.

Gastrocnemius ⑮

• Rest your ankle on your knee and repeat the same kneading massage movements on the calf muscles traveling upwards to the back of the knee.

• Repeat each complete leg sequence at least three times.

• Continue to foot massage of same leg.

Feet

The following movements ease the aches out of the feet, increase circulation, and generally tone up the whole body.

• With the foot resting on your thigh, hold the foot with the same — left or right — hand, resting the fingers of your other hand over the top of the foot. Use the thumb of that hand to make small circular movements traveling all over the instep and sole of your foot, paying particular attention to the area around the fleshy part of the instep.

• To massage the toes use the same movement as you did on the fingers — small round movements, holding the toe between the thumb and fingers, massaging with a movement rather like rolling a marble between thumb and fingers. Do this on each toe, traveling up the toe, spending time on the joints if you wish.

• Now sweep up the whole leg with both hands using a long smooth firm massage movement.

• Repeat the complete leg and foot massage on the other side.

$\mathcal{C}$hapter 8

Essential Oil Profiles

$\mathcal{T}$he pages which follow give details on the most widely used and available essential oils. There are many other essential oils which have not been listed here because although very useful, they are not easily obtained by the non-professionals. The information is self-explanatory, except perhaps for the list under "Therapeutic Properties." A glossary of the terms used is thus provided here. Forgetting the glossary words for a moment and running your eye down the list of things that essential oils can do, you get a good idea of what essential oils are all about. These therapeutic properties are in some cases thought to be the result of the particular chemical structures within the particular essential oil, and in other cases they are more of a mystery. The supreme complexity of essential oils is in the process of being unraveled but we still have far to go. Some of what is known is explained after the glossary.

First, I list some of the essential oils which have been found to be useful in combating various microscopic organisms. The list relates to the essential oils in the profiles.

Antiseptic Essential Oils

Basil, bay, bergamot, benzoin, black pepper, cardamom, cedarwood, chamomile roman, cinnamon, clary sage, clove, eucalyptus citriodora, eucalyptus globulus, eucalyptus radiata, frankincense, geranium, grapefruit, hyacinth, jasmine, juniper, lavender, lemon, lemongrass, linden blossom, litsea cubeba, marjoram, melissa, myrrh, neroli, orange, oregano, ormenis flower, palmarosa, patchouli, peppermint, petitgrain, pine, ravensara, rose maroc, rosemary, rose otto, sandalwood, spikenard, tagetes, tea tree, thyme (red and linalol), vetiver, ylang ylang, yuzu

---

Antibiotic Essential Oils

Basil, bay, bergamot, cinnamon, clove, eucalyptus radiata, frankincense, geranium, lavender, lemon, litsea cubeba, manuka, melissa, oregano, patchouli, ravensara, spikenard, tagetes, tea tree, thyme (red and linalol), yuzu

---

Anti-Fungal Essential Oils

Cedarwood, clove, eucalyptus citriodora, manuka, myrrh, patchouli, spikenard, tagetes, tea tree, yuzu

---

Anti-Viral Essential Oils

Cinnamon, clove, eucalyptus radiata, melissa, oregano, ravensara, tea tree, thyme (red and linalol)

Anti-Infectious Essential Oils

Chamomile roman, clary sage, clove, eucalyptus globulus, eucalyptus radiata, geranium, grapefruit, lavender, lemon, lemongrass, marjoram, neroli, ormenis flower, palmarosa, patchouli, peppermint, pine, ravensara, rose maroc, rose otto, sandalwood, spikenard, tagetes, tea tree, thyme (red and linalol), yuzu

---

Glossary of the Therapeutic Uses of Essential Oils

Analgesic: reduces pain sensation

Antibiotic/antibacterial: prevents bacterial growth

Anti-fungal: prevents fungal growth

Anti-infectious: prevents uptake of infection

Anti-parasitic: acts against insect parasites

Anti-putrescent: acts against putrefaction

Antisclerotic: prevents hardening of cells and tissues

Antiseptic: destroys microbes and prevents their development

Anti-spasmodic: prevents or relieves spasms, convulsions, or contractions

Anti-sudorific: prevents sweating

Antitussive: relieves coughs

Anti-viral: prevents viral growth

Balsamic: soothes sore throats, coughs, etc.

Calmative: sedative, calming agent

Carminative: relieves flatulence, easing abdominal pain and bloating

Cholagogue: promotes the evacuation of bile from gall bladder and ducts

Cicatrisive: promotes the formation of scar tissue, thus healing

Cytophylactic: promotes cell turnover, thus healing

Depurative: cleanser, detoxifier; purifies blood and internal organs

Diuretic: promotes the removal of excess water from the body by urine

Emmenagogue: induces or regularizes menstruation

Emollient: soothes and softens skin

Expectorant: promotes removal of mucus from the body

Febrifuge: an anti-febrile (anti-fever) agent

Galactagogue: induces the flow of milk

Haemostatic: stops bleeding

Hepatic: acts on the liver

Immunostimulant: stimulates the action of the immune system

Mucolytic: breaks down mucous

Nervine: acts on nerves; relieves nervous disorders

Pectoral: beneficial for diseases or conditions of the chest and respiratory system

Rubefacient: a counter-irritant producing redness of the skin

Sedative: reduces mental excitement or physical activity

Soporific: induces, or tends to induce, sleep

Stimulant: increases overall function of the body

Stomachic: good for the stomach; gastric tonic, digestive aid

Tonic: invigorates, refreshes, and restores bodily functions

Vermifuge: expels intestinal worms

Vulnerary: heals wounds and sores by external application

The Chemistry of Essential Oils

When essential oils are analyzed by gas chromatography or other means, the machine produces a graph which translates into a list of perhaps one or two hundred naturally occurring chemical constituents. In terms of these constituents, each essential oil is different. There are several main types of constituent groupings, including hydrocarbons, esters, aldehydes, ketones, and phenols. For example, under the general heading of "alcohols" one might find linalol, citronellol, geraniol, or T-Cadinol, among others, while under "phenols" there might be eugenol, thymol, and cavracrol. A certain amount is known about the therapeutic action of some of these constituents, both in terms of the larger groupings and the individual components. For example, the phenols have been shown to have an anti-microbial action while citronellol, which is an alcohol, has been shown to have sedative properties.

For the interested reader I provide some information regarding the connection between chemical groupings found in essential oils, and the therapeutic properties attributed to them. When looking for an essential oil to do a particular job, such as to fight inflammation, one might look for essential oils that contain particular acids and alderhydes. If the desired effect is a sedative, one might look for essential oils containing certain types of aldehydes, ethers, alcohols, coumarins, and esters.

Another way to look at essential oils is to look at

their electro-positive or electro-negative charge. For example, phenols have a positive charge which is said by some to partly explain the fact that phenols are generally warming and strengthening; while alderhydes have a negative charge and are thought to be cooling and calming. This kind of analysis, however, cannot be definitive. An essential oil is more than the sum of its parts and has to be considered as a whole, so although the main component may in fact be electro-positive, that does not tell us whether the entire essential oil — in conjunction with its many other components — still has this quality, because not enough research has been done in this area.

Being made of so many components — sometimes as many as three hundred — essential oils are very complex and it cannot be said that the main component or even the two or three most prevalent components account for an essential oil's particular therapeutic characteristics. It is all the components working in synergistic harmony that makes an essential oil what it is, not one particular chemical within it.

Also, many essential oils are "adaptogenic," meaning they can have either a stimulant or sedative action, depending upon the physiological and psychological condition of the person they are being applied to. It is this "balancing" nature which truly reflects the subtle, but positive, nature of essential oils.

Acids: anti-inflammatory, stimulant

Alcohols: energizing, stimulating, circulation stimulant, toning, general tonic, nerve tonic — uplifting, hypotensive, antibacterial, vitalizing, sedative, hypnotic, narcotic effect, balancing

Aldehydes: anti-infectious, anti-inflammatory, calming, relaxing, sedative, soothing, cooling, nerve tonic — uplifting, hypnotic

Coumarins: calming, sedative, hypnotic, hypotensive, nerve tonic, relaxing

Esters: anti-spasmodic, sedative, calming, relaxing, hypotensive, balancing, soothing, general tonic, nerve tonic — uplifting, cooling

Ethers: anti-infectious, anti-spasmodic, calming, relaxing, sedative, analgesic, balancing, soothing, stimulating

Hydrocarbons: cooling, calming

Ketones: stimulating, mucolytic agent, calming, nerve tonic — uplifting

Lactones: calming, relaxing

Monoterpenes: stimulating, warming

Monoterpenols: stimulating, warming

Oxides: stimulating, warming

Phenols: anti-spasmodic, anti-infectious, vaso-constrictor, anti-microbial, immunostimulant, general stimulant, general tonic, nerve tonic — uplifting, warming, stimulating, strengthening

Sesquiterpenes: anti-spasmodic, calming, relaxing, general tonic

Terpenes: anti-infectious, vaso-decongestant, stimulant, general tonic, warming

| BASIL | Latin name: *Ocimum basilicum* |

Family species: *Labiatae*

Purchasing guide: Color: Pale yellow; **Viscosity:** Watery; **Aroma:** Warm, rich, fiery, sharp, peppery, aniseed-like

Countries of origin: Egypt, Comore Islands (Madagascar), France, USA, Italy, Spain, Vietnam

Description: Annual herb growing up to three feet high. The flowers are white-ish to pink-ish, depending on species.

Part used: Leaves and flowering tops

Extraction method: Steam distillation

Yield: 0.1–0.2%

Most valuable uses: Weak nervous conditions, mental fatigue, headaches, tension, stress, muscular spasm, concentration, physical and mental sluggishness

Therapeutic properties: Restorative, general stimulant, anti-spasmodic, emmenagogic, stomachic, digestive tonic, intestinal antiseptic, carminative, anti-infectious, antibiotic

Main chemical components: Phenol Methylchavicol, Linalol, Eugenol, Cineol, Pinene, Camphor

Blends well with: Bergamot, black pepper, cedarwood, chamomile roman, clary sage, coriander, cypress, eucalyptus (all), fennel, geranium, ginger, grapefruit, juniper, lavender, lemon, marjoram, niaouli, orange, oregano, palmarosa, pine, rosemary, sage, tea tree, thyme linalol

Interesting facts: Derived from the Greek word for "king," *basileus*. In Ayurvedic medicine is called tulsi. Considered a holy herb in India, sacred to Krishna and Vishnu. Became the protective plant of the house, and spirit of the family. It is said that every good Hindu places a basil leaf on his/her chest when resting. Also associated with scorpions — perhaps because the oil can prickle when in direct contact with the skin.

Contraindications: Not to be used during pregnancy. Can cause irritation to sensitive skin. Should not be used on children under 16 years of age. Not to be used in baths.

BAY — Latin name: *Pimenta racemosa*

Family species: *Myrtaceae*

Purchasing guide: Color: Deep yellow; **Viscosity:** Medium to watery; **Aroma:** Spicy, sweet, fresh, balsamic. *Not to be confused with Laurel Leaf Oil* (Laurus nobilis).

Countries of origin: St. Thomas (Virgin Islands), Jamaica, South and Central America

Description: A small evergreen tree growing to 25 feet high with small branches bearing strongly aromatic leaves and small white flowers forming a flower head.

Part used: Leaves collected from five-year-old (minimum) shrubs

Extraction method: Steam distillation (often salt is added, or sea water is used in the still)

Yield: 0.5–1.5%

Most valuable uses: Rheumatism, muscular pain, neuralgia, circulation, colds, flu, calming, dental infections, diarrhea, skin infections, general fatigue

Therapeutic properties: Antiseptic, antibiotic, analgesic, anti-neuralgic, anti-infectious, general stimulant, hypertensive

Main chemical components: Eugenol, Chavicol, Myrcene, Cineol, Methyl eugenol

Blends well with: Benzoin, bergamot, black pepper, cardamom, cinnamon, clove, coriander, frankincense, geranium, ginger, lavender, grapefruit, lemon, mandarin, nutmeg, orange, petitgrain, rosemary, sandalwood, ylang ylang

Interesting facts: The bay tree is used medicinally. In the past, the leaves were distilled with rum, which is the source of bay rum, a famous hair tonic and body rub for colds, muscle pains, etc.

Contraindications: Use in moderation.

BENZOIN   Latin name: *Styrax benzoin dryander*

Family species: *Styraceae*

Purchasing guide: Color: Golden brown;
Viscosity: Viscous, treacle-like; **Aroma:** Warm,
balsamic, chocolately-vanilla.
*Not to be confused with other benzoin species
which are used by the perfume trade.*

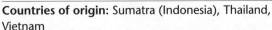

Countries of origin: Sumatra (Indonesia), Thailand,
Vietnam

Description: Birch-like tree growing to 20 feet high,
producing white sap which becomes hard and brittle, and
yellowish-brown in color. The tree grows rapidly but is only
"worked" after seven years. The bark is deliberately cut,
causing the sap to run, and it is collected from the bark.

Part used: Resin

Extraction method: Solvent extraction

Yield: 65–85%

Most valuable uses: Catarrh, bronchitis, coughs, colds,
wounds, acne, eczema, psoriasis, ulcerations, rheumatism,
arthritis, scar tissue, circulation, muscular stiffness, nervous
tension, stress, emotional crisis

Therapeutic properties: Antiseptic, antidepressant,
vulnerary, expectorant, pectoral

Main chemical components: Benzoic Acid, Benzyl
Benzoate, Benzyl Alcohol, Vanillin, Coniferyl benzoate

Blends well with: Bay, bergamot, black pepper, cardamom, clary sage, coriander, frankincense, ginger, geranium, grapefruit, lemon, litsea cubeba, jasmine, marjoram,
niaouli, nutmeg, orange, patchouli, palmarosa, rose maroc,
rose otto, sandalwood, vetiver, ylang ylang

Interesting facts: There are four varieties of benzoin tree,
and oil, although only *styrax benzoin dryander* is used medicinally, the others being used in perfumery. The species
described here was discovered in 1787 by Jonas Dryander.
The oil is an ingredient of Friar's Balsam.

Contraindications: Possible irritant to sensitive skin.

BERGAMOT Latin name: *Citrus aurantium ssp bergamia*

Family species: *Rutaceae*

Purchasing guide: Color: Green to yellow; **Viscosity:** Watery; **Aroma:** Sweet, fruity, fresh citrus with spicy floral undertones

Countries of origin: Italy (Reggio di Calabria) — where 90% of the world's crop is produced. Also Ivory Coast, Morocco, Tunisia, and Algeria.

Description: A tree growing to 13 or more feet, with white star-shaped flowers. Some branches have thorns. Bearing a citrus fruit, resembling a cross between an orange and a grapefruit, green turning yellow in color.

Part used: Rind of both ripe and unripe fruit

Extraction method: Cold expression

Yield: 0.5% of fresh fruit rind

Most valuable uses: Depression, stress, tension, fear, hysteria, infection (all types including skin), anorexia, psoriasis, nervous eczema, emotional crisis, convalescence.

Therapeutic properties: Antiseptic, antibiotic, anti-spasmodic, stomachic, antidepressant, calmative, febrifuge, vermifuge

Main chemical components: D Limonene, Linalyl Acetate, Linalol, gamma Terpinene, Bergaptene

Blends well with: All essential oils, including: black pepper, clary sage, cypress, frankincense, geranium, helichrysum, jasmine, lavender, mandarin, nutmeg, orange, ormenis flower, rosemary, sandalwood, vetiver, ylang ylang

Interesting facts: The name comes from the northern Italian town of Bergamo, near Milan, the first main trade center. Introduced into Italy in 1600 from Pergamum, now called Bergama, in Turkey. Used as flavorant in Earl Grey tea. The green tint is due to the chlorophyll content. Widely used in eau de colognes.

Contraindications: Not to be used neat on the skin. Not to be applied to the skin (even in diluted form) before exposure to the sun. Bergamot contains bergaptene, which is known to be phototoxic (increases the effect of sunlight).

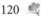

BLACK PEPPER Latin name: *Piper nigrum*

Family species: *Piperaceae*

Purchasing guide: Color: Greenish-yellow to yellow-ish-white; **Viscosity:** Watery; **Aroma:** Strong, warm, and peppery

Countries of origin: India, Malaysia, Madagascar, China, Indonesia

Description: A climbing woody vine, like bindweed, with a life of about 20 years. The vine clings to trees for support and shade. It has small white flowers which produce the fruit of red berries.

Part used: Unripe fruit/berry

Extraction method: Steam distillation

Yield: 2%

Most valuable uses: Pain-relief, digestive problems, rheumatism, chills, flu, coughs, colds, increases circulation, exhaustion, muscular aches, physical and emotional coldness, nerve tonic, fevers

Therapeutic properties: Analgesic, antiseptic, expectorant, tonic, febrifuge, aphrodisiac, anti-catarrhal, digestive, moderate rubefacient, diuretic

Main chemical components: A-Pinene, B-Pinene, Sabinene, Limonene, beta Caryophyllene, Camphene

Blends well with: Bergamot, clary sage, clove, coriander, fennel, frankincense, geranium, ginger, grapefruit, lavender, juniper, lemon, lemongrass, lime, mandarin, marjoram, myrrh, orange, nutmeg, patchouli, palmarosa, rosemary, spikenard, sage, sandalwood, tea tree, valerian, vetiver, ylang ylang

Interesting facts: Used in India for over 4,000 years. Known to have been used in Chinese medicine, and by the ancient Greeks. It featured in the spice wars as a trading commodity. There are over 900 species of pepper but only about ten are used in medicines.

Contraindications: May cause redness on sensitive skin.

CARDAMOM   Latin name: *Elettaria cardamomum Maton*

Family species: *Zingiberaceae*

Purchasing guide: **Color:** Clear to pale yellow; **Viscosity:** Medium watery; **Aroma:** Fresh, sweet green, spicy, balsamic

Countries of origin: India (Malabar Coast), Sri Lanka, Tanzania, Guatemala

Description: Perennial herb of the rush-like type, with blade type leaves, small yellow flowers with violet tips, and seed-bearing fruit.

Part used: Seeds of the fruit. Green fruit capsules have the most essential oil.

Extraction method: Steam distillation

Yield: 1–5%

Most valuable uses: Indigestion, flatulence, mental fatigue, water retention, muscular cramps, muscular spasms, stomach cramps, physical exhaustion, catarrh, sinus headaches, constipation

Therapeutic properties: Antiseptic, digestive stimulant, calmative, stomachic, diuretic, anti-spasmodic, expectorant

Main chemical components: Alpha Terpinyl Acetate, 1,8, Cineole, Terpinen-4-ol, Alpha-terpineol, Sabinene, Limonene

Blends well with: Bay, bergamot, black pepper, cedarwood, cinnamon, clover, coriander, fennel, ginger, grapefruit, lemon, lemongrass, mandarin, litsea cubeba, neroli, orange, patchouli, palmarosa, petitgrain, sandalwood, vetiver, ylang ylang, jasmine

Interesting facts: There are many varieties, some of which were known to the Greeks and Romans. The essential oil was first distilled in 1544 by Valerius Cordus, following a Portuguese explorer's procuring them from the southwest Indian coast. The Arabs use cardamom in coffee, especially as hospitality, while in Scandinavian countries it is used in liqueurs. Cardamom is a well-known and important ingredient in Asian cooking.

Contraindications: None known.

CARNATION   Latin name: *Dianthus caryophyllus*

Family species: *Caryophyllaceae*

Purchasing guide: Color: Brown; **Viscosity:** Medium to viscous; **Aroma:** Rich, floral, spicy, honey-clove.

Bay essential oil and synthetic aromatics such as eugenol, isoeugenol, and phenyl ethyl alcohol are sometimes used to adulterate carnation oil. Only very small amounts of absolute oil are used in blends as these oils can be very strong.

Countries of origin: France, Egypt

Description: Perennial herb, with greyish-green, long slender leaves, growing from the stem. The pink flowers have many petals which have a ragged edge. Where the petal joins the center, some types have slight flecks of darker pink to purple on them.

Part used: Flower heads

Extraction method: Solvent extraction then alcohol extraction which produces an absolute

Yield: 0.05%

Most valuable uses: Used in aroma-psychology, such as emotional problems, stress, feelings of detachment, overactive mind, inability to communicate, emotional solitude, feeling neglected

Therapeutic properties: Calmative, sedative, neurotonic, soporific

Main chemical components: Eugenol, B-Caryophyllene, Caryophyllene Oxide

Blends well with: Rose maroc, rose otto, clove, lemon, black pepper, bergamot, lemon, orange, neroli, ylang ylang, sandalwood, jasmine, clary sage, chamomile roman, coriander, cardamom, hyacinth, vetiver, yuzu

Interesting facts: This type of carnation is also known as "pinks" due to the color of the flower. Although this oil is quite difficult to find, there are a few retail companies who sell it. The name may derive from the fact that the flower was woven into ancient garlands and crowns, hence carnation. Symbolic of divine love and said to bring luck. It takes 500 kilograms of flowers to make one kg of concrete which, in turn, yields 100 grams of absolute.

Contraindications: None known.

CEDARWOOD   Latin name: *Cedrus atlantica*

Family species: *Pinaceae (pine)*

Purchasing guide: Color: Pale yellow to light orange; **Viscosity:** Viscous to semi-solid; **Aroma:** Balsamic, soft, woody, sweet, warm. *Several different types of essential oils are distilled from other species of cedar, for example,* Juniperas virginiana *and* Cedrus libani *(Himalayan cedar). Not to be confused with leaf oil distilled from the Northern White Cedar* (Thuja occidentalis) *which has been reported to be toxic and dangerous.*

Countries of origin: Morocco, Algeria, USA, China

Description: An evergreen tree with wide branches tapering to a height of 50 feet. The branches are covered with long needles, having barrel-shaped cones. Some of the cedars in Lebanon, however, are said to be 100 feet high and over 2,000 years old.

Part used: Wood chips and sawdust

Extraction method: Steam distillation

Yield: 3.5%

Most valuable uses: Chest infections, urinary infections, acne, general tonic, cleansing, rheumatism, asthma, anxiety, cystitis, scalp disorders, cellulite

Therapeutic properties: Antiseptic, tonic, anti-fungal, anti-seborrheic, regenerative

Main chemical components: Alpha & Beta Cedrene, Cedrol, Atlantone, Caryophyllene, Cadinene

Blends well with: Bay, bergamot, cardamom, chamomile roman, clary sage, cypress, eucalyptus (all), frankincense, geranium, grapefruit, juniper, lavender, marjoram, orange, neroli, palmarosa, petitgrain, rosemary, sandalwood, ylang ylang

Interesting facts: Repellent to insects. Used by the ancient Egyptians for mummification and by other ancient cultures for sarcophagi and palace and temple building material. Sometimes called "satin wood." Latin name means "Atlas cedar," the tree growing in the Atlas Mountains that span Morocco and Algeria. Different species of cedars are found all over the world. Native Americans use cedar as medicine and burn it for purification.

Contraindications: Not to be used during pregnancy (especially if using the species *Juniperas virginiana*). Not to be used by children under 18 years.

CHAMOMILE GERMAN   Latin name: *Matricaria chamomilla*

Family species: *Asteraceae* (formerly placed in the Compositae family)

Purchasing guide: Color: Dark blue; **Viscosity:** Medium; **Aroma:** Sweet, straw-like and herby. *Sometimes adulterated with juniper tar oil.*

Countries of origin: France, Morocco, Spain, Hungary, Egypt, Iran, Afghanistan, Balkans, South America

Description: Annual herbaceous plant growing to 40 inches with white flowers with hollow, yellow conical-shaped centers.

Part used: Flowering tops

Extraction method: Steam distillation

Yield: 0.2–0.4% of fresh flowering tops

Most valuable uses: Inflammation, menstrual disorders, skin problems including rashes, asthma, eczema, rheumatism, arthritis, acne, chilblains, ulcerations, muscular spasms

Therapeutic properties: Calmative, analgesic, anti-spasmodic, antibiotic, febrifuge, anti-inflammatory, immunostimulant, emmenagogue, digestive, hepatic, vulnerary

Main chemical components: Alpha Bisabolol, Chamazulene, Bisabolol Oxide, Farnesene, En-yn-dicycloether

Blends well with: Bergamot, chamomile roman, lavender, cypress, frankincense, geranium, benzoin, marjoram, lemon, grapefruit, naiouli, patchouli, pine, ravensara, rosemary, tea tree

Interesting facts: The name "Matricaria" comes from the Latin *matrix,* meaning "womb," because of its widespread use by women for gynecological conditions. Used in French liqueurs and for flavoring tobacco.

Contraindications: None known.

CHAMOMILE ROMAN   Latin name: *Anthemis nobilis*

Family species: *Asteraceae* (formerly placed in the Compositae family)

Purchasing guide: Color: clear blue; **Viscosity:** watery; **Aroma:** fruity, sweet, fresh, herbaceous, rather apple-like

Countries of origin: England, Bulgaria, France, Hungary, Italy, Chile

Description: Plant grows 20 inches high with green feathery leaves and small white flowers with yellow centers, growing on strong stems.

Part used: Flowers

Extraction method: Steam distillation

Yield: 1.7% from fresh flower heads. (The distillation of dried calices — the part left after the petals fall off — produces a yellow oil which may not have the same properties as true flower chamomile roman, which should always be blue)

Most valuable uses: Pain-relief, fevers, menstrual problems, skin problems such as rashes, eczema, chilblains, teething pain and other children's ailments, muscular spasms, sedative, rheumatism, depression, nervousness

Therapeutic properties: Analgesic, anti-spasmodic, calmative, antiseptic, antibiotic, anti-inflammatory, anti-infectious, vulnerary, immunostimulant, sedative, anti-neuralgic, nervine, antidepressant

Main chemical components: Esters of Angelic, Butyric & Tiglic Acids, Bisabolol, Farnesol

Blends well with: Lavender, geranium, lemon, tea tree, eucalyptus, palmarosa, grapefruit, rose otto, neroli, jasmine, clary sage

Interesting facts: The Latin name derives from the Greek word *anthemis*, meaning "little flower." Used for flavoring fine French liqueurs. The blue azulen content is created during the distillation process. For over 2,000 years it has been used extensively as a medicine. In ancient Egypt and early Scandinavian culture chamomile was associated with the sun god.

Contraindications: None known.

CINNAMON   Latin name: *Cinnamomum zeylanicum*

Family species: *Lauraceae*

Purchasing guide: Color: Yellow (leaf oil); brownish-red (bark oil); **Viscosity:** Medium to watery; **Aroma:** Warm, spicy, sweet, smoky

Countries of origin: Sri Lanka, India, Madagascar and Comores, Seychelles

Description: Evergreen tree which can grow to 20–30 feet high but cultivated as a bush, with thick bark, greenish-orange speckled shoots, small white flowers and fruit which, when ripe, becomes bluish with white spots.

Part used: Leaves and twigs (inner dried bark)

Extraction method: Steam distillation (both)

Yield: 1.6–1.8% (bark: 0.5–1%)

Most valuable uses: Infections, coughs, colds, flu, rheumatism, arthritis, general debility, aches, pains

Therapeutic properties: Stimulant, antiseptic, antibiotic, anti-viral, anti-putrescent, analgesic, anti-spasmodic, emmenagogue

Main chemical components: Eugenol, beta Caryophyllene, Linalool, Methyl chavicol

Blends well with: Clove, nutmeg, ylang ylang, mandarin, orange, lemon, grapefruit, benzoin, litsea cubeba, rose maroc, bay, bergamot, carnation, coriander, cardamom, frankincense, geranium, ginger, lemongrass, marjoram, patchouli, pettitgrain, yuzu

Interesting facts: The tree/bush grows well in nearly pure sand. The dried bark is extensively used as a spice in food flavoring. Essential oils can be extracted from all parts — bark, leaves, stem and root — all being slightly different. The word "cinnamon" is taken from the Greek word *kinnamon,* meaning tube or pipe, indicating the appearance of the bark used as a spice.

Contraindications: Not to be used in pregnancy. Not to be used on children under 18. Not to be used by people with sensitive skin. Not to be used in baths. Only use in low doses. Best used in blends in the diffuser methods.

CLARY SAGE   Latin name: *Salvia sclarea*

Family species: *Lamiaceae* (or *Labiatae*)

Purchasing guide: **Color:** Colorless to pale yellow; **Viscosity:** Watery (only viscous if the leaves are included in distillation — when the color can be greenish); **Aroma:** nutty, warm, light, musky, herbaceous

Countries of origin: France, Spain, Bulgaria, Russia, Italy, USA, England, Morocco, Germany

Description: Biennial plant growing up to 3 feet high with large hairy leaves which only grow to half the height of the plant. The lilac-pink flowers rise above the leaves, coming directly off long, thin stems.

Part used: Flowering tops

Extraction method: Steam distillation

Yield: 0.3 to 1%, depending on crop

Most valuable uses: Muscular fatigue, menstrual problems, PMS, fertility, exhaustion, insomnia, menopausal problems, calming, stress, depression, cramps, excessive perspiration

Therapeutic properties: Antiseptic, calmative, tonic, emmenagogue, anti-infectious, anti-spasmodic, anti-sudorific, aphrodisiac, nerve tonic, nervine, estrogen-like

Main chemical components: Linalol, Linalyl Acetate, Germacrene, Geranyl acetate

Blends well with: Geranium, lemon, grapefruit, lavender, sandalwood, cypress, mandarin, jasmine, juniper, rose maroc, rose otto, bergamot, bay, black pepper, chamomile roman, coriander, lime, patchouli, tea tree. Blends well with most flower absolutes in small dosages.

Interesting facts: The name "salvia" is derived from the Latin word for "good health." In Germany, the herb was used, with elderflowers as an additive to cheap wine to make it taste like Muscatel. Also used to flavor vermouths and liqueurs. In Britain, it's used as a substitute for hops in beer making. In Jamaica, the plant was blended with coconut to ease scorpion stings. The seeds were used in many countries to clear conditions of the eye — hence the name "clear-eye."

Contraindications: Avoid during pregnancy.

CLOVE   Latin name: *Eugenia caryophyllata*

Family species: Myrtaceae

Purchasing guide: Color: Pale yellow; **Viscosity:** Medium to watery; **Aroma:** Rich, warm, sweet, spicy
A different oil, clove leaf oil, has a harsh odor and is darker in color and should not be used in aromatherapy.

Countries of origin: Indonesia, Madagascar, Sri Lanka, Tanzania, West Indies

Description: An evergreen tree, growing to a height of between 40–50 feet, with large bright green leaves. At the end of the twigs the strongly fragrant flowers grow in bunches. The buds turn from green to a rose-peach which, upon drying, turns into a deep red brown.

Part used: Two essential oils are distilled, one from the leaves, which is not used in aromatherapy, and one from the sundried buds

Extraction method: Steam distillation

Yield: 10–15%

Most valuable uses: Warts, verrucas, toothache, muscle pain, tired limbs, rheumatism, colds, flu, stress, mental debility, diarrhea, chest infections, bronchitis, nausea, scabies, ringworm, general exhaustion, recovery from infections

Therapeutic properties: Antiseptic, antibiotic, anti-viral, antifungal, stimulant, analgesic, anti-neuralgic, anti-spasmodic, carminative, aphrodisiac, anti-infectious, stomachic, tonic, antiparasitic

Main chemical components: Eugenol, Acetoeugenol, Eugenyl Acetate, Caryophyllene, d-cadinene

Blends well with: Lemon, geranium, lavender, grapefruit, chamomile roman, ginger, palmarosa, ylang ylang, sandalwood, mandarin, jasmine, clary sage, bay, benzoin

Interesting facts: Clove was used in ancient China as medicine. To fragrance their mouths the courtiers would hold clove buds in their mouths when speaking to the emperors. The Romans prized clove as food flavoring and as medicine, recognizing it as an important aspect of spice trade. It is still used in dental preparations as it has slight analgesic action. Used extensively in cooking, soap and perfumery; often used in pomades stuck in oranges; and used in mulled wines and liqueurs.

Contraindications: May cause skin irritation on sensitive skin. Avoid during pregnancy. Do not use on children under 12 years. Do not use in baths.

| CORIANDER | Latin name: *Coriandrum sativum* |

Family species: *Apiaceae* or *Umbelliferae*

Purchasing guide: Color: Colorless to pale yellow; **Viscosity:** Watery; **Aroma:** Sweet, warm, spicy

Countries of origin: India, Egypt, Russia, France, Morocco, Tunisia, Italy, USA, Romania

Description: Annual or biennial plant, between one to three feet high with sparse, fine, spindly leaves, delicate whitish-pink flowers, followed by green seeds.

Part used: Seeds

Extraction method: Steam distillation from crushed ripe seeds

Yield: 0.8–1.0%

Most valuable uses: Digestive problems, flatulence, stomach cramps, aches due to fatigue, mental fatigue, rheumatism

Therapeutic properties: Sedative, anti-spasmodic, carminative, stimulant, tonic, stomachic, depurative, regenerative

Main chemical components: Linalol, Limonene, gamma Terpinene, Geraniol, Carvone

Blends well with: Bergamot, clary sage, black pepper, cardamom, cinnamon, clove, cypress, frankincense, geranium, ginger, grapefruit, lemon, neroli, nutmeg, orange, palmarosa, petitgrain, pine, ravensara, sandalwood, vetiver, ylang ylang, jasmine

Interesting facts: Coriander seeds have been used for thousands of years. They were found in Tutankhamun's tomb. Coriander seeds are used to flavor the famous Chartreuse and Benedictine liqueurs that are still made by monks in France.

Contraindications: None known.

CYPRESS   Latin name: *Cupressus sempervirens*

Family species: *Conifera* or *Cupressaceae*

Purchasing guide: Color: Colorless to slightly yellow; **Viscosity:** Watery; **Aroma:** Woody, warm, slightly spicy

Country of origin: France, Spain

Description: Cone-shaped evergreen tree growing to 80 feet, with dark green foliage and cones, which have seed-nuts inside.

Part used: Foliage and twigs of young branches

Extraction method: Steam distillation

Yield: 1.3–1.5%

Most valuable uses: Circulation, varicose veins, hemor-rhoids, menopausal problems, menstrual problems, coughs, asthma and some other respiratory problems, fluid reten-tion, cellulite, rheumatism, tension, nervousness

Therapeutic properties: Astringent, anti-spasmodic, anti-sudorific, diuretic, restorative, cicatrisive, vasoconstrictor, respiratory tonic, calmative

Main chemical components: Alpha Pinene, delta 3 Carene, Myrcene, Cedrol, Cedrine, Terpinolene, Limonene

Blends well with: Bergamot, clary sage, lemon, lavender, orange, lime, juniper, pine, marjoram, chamomile roman, mandarin, sandalwood, rosemary, geranium, eucalyptus (all), frankincense, cedarwood, pine, ravensara, rosemary, tea tree

Interesting facts: The tree gave its name to the island of Cyprus. The cross of Jesus is thought to have been made of cypress. The Chinese consider the nuts to be beneficial to the liver. Associated with burial grounds and, hence, grief. The wood is impervious to woodworm, making it useful for works of art and furniture.

Contraindications: None known.

EUCALYPTUS CITRIODORA   Latin name: *Eucalyptus citriodora* **(Lemon Eucalyptus)**

Family species: *Myrtaceae*

Purchasing guide: Color: Clear to light yellow; **Viscosity:** Watery; **Aroma:** Strong, balsamic, lemony

Countries of origin: Australia, Brazil, China, India, South Africa

Description: Tall evergreen tree with white blotchy trunk and fluffy white flowers. In oil production, the tree is cut back to about five feet to encourage new growth, because most oil is concentrated in new leaves.

Part used: Leaves and twigs

Extraction method: Steam distillation

Yield: 2–2.4% (wild species 1%)

Most valuable uses: Chest infections, antiseptic, fungal infections, insect repellent, sores, wounds, asthma, sore throat, fever, chicken pox, measles, bacterial skin infections, general body tonic, rheumatism, relaxation, arthritis, cystitis

Therapeutic properties: Anti-infectious, antiseptic, anti-inflammatory, calmative, pectoral, antibiotic, vulnerary, anti-fungal

Main chemical components: Citronellal, Citronellyl Acetate, Citronellol, 1,8-cineole, Linalool

Blends well with: Basil, benzoin, black pepper, cedarwood, clary sage, clove, cypress, other eucalyptus oils, frankincense, geranium, ginger, juniper, lavender, marjoram, orange, peppermint, pine, ravensara, rosemary, sage, tea tree, thyme linalol, vetiver, ylang ylang

Interesting facts: Used as an insect repellent for cockroaches, silver fish, etc. The wood is used in situations requiring strength and flexibility, such as the bottom frame of carriages, ship building, bridge construction, flooring, handles of shovels and picks, etc. Used to be included in a three-variety eucalyptus cigarette on sale in Australia.

Contraindications: None known.

EUCALYPTUS GLOBULUS   Latin name: *Eucalyptus globulus*

Family species: *Myrtaceae*

Purchasing guide: **Color:** Clear to pale yellow; **Viscosity:** Watery; **Aroma:** Strong, woody, camphory. *The yellow color develops with age.*

Countries of origin: Australia, China, Portugal, Spain

Description: A tall tree with a smooth white bar, which can grow to over 100 feet, with long sliver-green, sickle-shaped leaves which often grow to nine inches in length. It has large, fluffy white flowers which grow from the fruit, a woody calyx, an enclosed cup-shape which contains the many seeds.

Part used: Leaves and twigs

Extraction method: Steam distillation

Yield: 1.8–2%

Most valuable uses: Catarrh, bronchitis, colds, flu, fever, sinusitis, muscular aches and pains, headaches, sluggishness, mental exhaustion, rheumatism, asthma, insect bites, rashes, skin ulcers, chilblains, sore throats

Therapeutic properties: Antiseptic, balsamic, expectorant, antibiotic, anti-fungal, febrifuge, anti-infectious, anti-parasitic, anti-neuralgic, anti-putrescent, pectoral. *The antiseptic properties of this oil increase with age.*

Main chemical components: 1,8-Cineole, para Cymene, Eucalyptol, Fenchene, Globulol, Camphene

Blends well with: Lavender, rosemary, chamomile roman, chamomile german, peppermint, thyme linalol, thyme red, lemon, grapefruit, geranium, ginger, juniper, cypress, pine

Interesting facts: Essential oil was first distilled in Australia in 1788 by the Surgeon General of the colony, Dr. John White. The tree is commonly known as the "Tasmanian Blue Gum." The international interest in the tree developed because it is very fast growing and uses up large amounts of water, thus being able to turn swamp into usable land. Probably because this process destroyed the breeding ground of the malaria mosquito, the tree gained a reputation in the 19th century of being able to rid a locale of "miasma" or "fever" when the source of the malaria was not yet known. Hence the name "fever tree." Sometimes called "Blue Gum Oil."

Contraindications: Not to be used on children under 12 years.

EUCALYPTUS RADIATA   Latin name: *Eucalyptus radiata*

Family species: *Myrtaceae*

Purchasing guide: **Color:** Clear; **Viscosity:** Watery; **Aroma:** Woody, camphory, with faint peppermint undertone

Country of origin: Australia

Description: Tall tree with hard black bark at lower part and smooth and white at the top, with lance-shaped, six-inch leaves, with a profusion of flowers growing from flat-topped calyx, the enclosed container for seeds.

Part used: Leaves and twigs

Extraction method: Steam distillation

Yield: 1.2–2%

Most valuable uses: Catarrh, bronchitis, colds, flu, fever, sinusitis, muscular aches and pains, headaches, sluggishness, mental exhaustion, rheumatism, asthma, insect bites, rashes, skin ulcers, chilblains, acne

Therapeutic properties: Antiseptic, anti-infectious, antibiotic, anti-viral, anti-inflammatory, expectorant, pectoral, vulnerary, tonic, febrifuge

Main chemical components: 1,8-Cineole, alpha-terpineol, limonene, alpha-pinene

Blends well with: Lavender, rosemary, chamomile roman, chamomile german, peppermint, thyme linalol, lemon, grapefruit, geranium, ginger, juniper, cypress, pine

Interesting facts: The tree is known as "White Top Peppermint" or "River White Gum." Its natural habitat is along river banks and coastal mountain ranges. The first known record of eucalyptus radiata distillation is 1898. Generally considered to be gentler than eucalyptus globulus.

Contraindications: None known.

FENNEL (Sweet)　　Latin name: *Foeniculum vulgare dulce*

Family species: *Umbelliferae*

Purchasing guide:　Color: Colorless to pale yellow;
Viscosity: Watery;　**Aroma:** Warm, sweet, aniseed-
like, peppery

Countries of origin: France, Germany, Italy,
Bulgaria, Hungary, Russia, India, Spain

Description: Biennial plant growing to 6 ½ feet, with
sparse bright green leaves, like delicate lace. The yellow flowers
are atop thin stalks, facing the sky in clusters and are replaced
by seeds.

Part used: Seeds

Extraction method: Steam distillation

Yield: 2–4% distillation of the crushed seeds

Most valuable uses: Abdominal pains or cramps, flatulence,
coughs, sore throats, digestive problems, menstrual problems,
PMS, menopausal problems, fertility, obesity, nausea, fluid
retention, liver problems

Therapeutic properties: Carminative, emmenagogue, estrogen-like, galactagogue, depurative, diuretic, stimulant, regenerative, anti-spasmodic, antiseptic, antibiotic, vermifuge, expectorant

Main chemical components: trans Anethole, Fenchone,
Estragol, Methylchavicol, Fenone, aplha-pinene

Blends well with: Juniper, geranium, lavender, bergamot,
black pepper, cardamom, cypress, ginger, grapefruit, lemon,
marjoram, niaouli, pine, ravensara, rosemary, sandalwood,
ylang-ylang

Interesting facts: Gives ozone into the atmosphere. Pliny
mentions 22 remedies containing fennel. Frequently mentioned
in Anglo-Saxon cooking and medicine. The ancient Greeks
thought it conveyed long life, courage, and strength. Their
name for fennel was *marathrion* from *maraino*, "meaning to
grow thin." Fennel's ability to stave off hunger was employed
during fasting days in Europe. It was consumed in large quantities in the household of Edward I of England in 1300 — 8½
pounds being sufficient for only one month's supply.

Contraindications: Do not use in pregnancy. Do not use on
babies, or on children under 16 years. Not to be used by people subject to epilepsy. Not to be used by people with high
estrogen levels. Not to be used by women with breast cancer.
Not to be used by people with kidney problems, including kidney stones.

FRANKINCENSE   Latin name: *Boswellia carterii*

Family species: *Burseraceae*

Purchasing guide: **Color:** Pale yellow;
Viscosity: Watery to slightly viscous; **Aroma:**
Warm, sweet, balsamic, spicy, incense-like

Countries of origin: Oman (plain of Dhofar),
Somalia, Ethiopia, Saudi Arabia

Description: Thorny shrub, with 21 alternating oval-
shaped leaflets, producing white or sometimes pink flowers
of five petals. The bark produces a resin when it is damaged
or deliberately cut, after about three months. This cut is
vertical, and at first a milky substance is exuded which, on
contact with air, then turns to the resin.

Part used: Oleoresin

Extraction method: Steam distillation

Yield: Up to 10%

Most valuable uses: Skin diseases or disorders, circulation
problems, hemorrhoids, coughs, colds, bronchitis, rheumatism, urinary tract infections, antiseptic, antibacterial,
depression, general tonic, mental fatigue

Therapeutic properties: Tonic, stimulant, expectorant,
cicatrisive, pectoral, antidepressant, balsamic, antiseptic,
revitalizer

Main chemical components: Alpha Pinene, beta Pinene,
Olibanol, Octyl acetate

Blends well with: Cypress, orange, mandarin, sandalwood,
vetiver, pine, geranium, lavender, neroli, bergamot, rose
maroc, rose otto, clary sage, coriander, grapefruit, lemon,
patchouli, palmarosa, ylang ylang

Interesting facts: Given to Jesus by a wise king, on the
occasion of his birth in Bethlehem. Used in the incense used
by Roman Catholic and Greek Orthodox churches. Frankincense is sometimes called Olibanum. Can grow without
soil. Important to the perfume trade.

Contraindications: None known.

GERANIUM	Latin names: *Pelargonium graveolens, P roseum, P asperum*

Family species: *Geraniaceae*

Purchasing guide: **Color:** Colorless to light green; **Viscosity:** Watery; **Aroma:** Flowery rose, sweet, soft, green

Countries of origin: Reunion (for Bourbon geranium), Madagascar, Egypt, Algeria, Morocco, Russia, China, France, USA

Description: Can grow to three feet high with rather sparse small leaves and small pinkish-white flowers.

Part used: Leaves and stalks

Extraction method: Steam distillation

Yield: 0.1–0.2%

Most valuable uses: Female reproductive disorders, fertility, circulatory disorders, antidepressant, menopause, bruising, ulceration, hemorrhoids, antibacterial, anti-infectious, nervous fatigue, emotional balance

Therapeutic properties: Astringent, haemostatic, diuretic, antiseptic, antidepressant, regenerative, tonic, antibiotic, anti-spasmodic, anti-infectious

Main chemical components: Citronellol, Geraniol, Citronellyl Formate, Linalol, Terpineol, iso menthone

Blends well with: Lemon, grapefruit, lavender, rosemary, chamomile roman, peppermint, clove, clary sage, ginger, palmarosa, ylang ylang, sandalwood, mandarin, juniper, cypress, benzoin, bergamot, black pepper, fennel, frankincense, orange, rose maroc, rose otto, jasmine

Interesting facts: Introduced into Europe from Africa in the 17th century. There are approximately 700 varieties of geranium, only about 10 of which supply essential oil. The ornamental type of geranium, known to gardeners, does not usually yield essential oil. Geranium is sometimes called "lemon plant." The essential oil is widely used in soap manufacture, and perfumery. The unique rose-like aroma is captured by harvesting just as the leaves turn yellow; previous to this, the aroma is more lemony.

Contraindications: None known.

GINGER	Latin name: *Zingiberaceae officinale*

Family species: *Zingiberacae*

Purchasing guide: Color: Pale yellow to amber; **Viscosity:** Medium to watery; **Aroma:** Characteristic of ginger

Countries of origin: India, Sri Lanka, China, Java, West Indies

Description: Perennial herb growing to over four feet high. Long lance-shaped leaves extend from a central stalk, atop of which the flowers grow — yellow with purple claws. The stalk grows from a rhizome, the roots extending downward.

Part used: Fresh or dried rhizome

Extraction method: Steam distillation

Yield: approx. 2–4%

Most valuable uses: Fractures, rheumatism, arthritis, numbness, muscle fatigue, digestive problems, nausea, colds and flu, emotional coldness, nervous exhaustion, general debility, sexual tonic, sea sickness

Therapeutic properties: Antiseptic, stimulant, stomachic, analgesic, carminative, aphrodisiac, fortifying, febrifuge, expectorant

Main chemical components: alpha & beta Zingiberene, ar Curcumene, Camphene, Neral, B-bisabolene

Blends well with: Lemon, grapefruit, geranium, sandalwood, palmarosa, mandarin, ylang ylang, juniper, eucalyptus (all), clove, rose maroc, neroli, jasmine, frankincense, vetiver, patchouli, cedarwood, coriander, lime, orange, bergamot

Interesting facts: Long known as an aphrodisiac in China, India, and elsewhere. In Senegal, West Africa, the women make belts with the rhizome, in the hope of arousing their partner's sexual interest. Used for making ginger beer, ginger wine, and candy. Used in ancient Chinese and Indian Ayurvedic medicine. Much sought after in ancient times. Oil used in perfumery changes the aroma of a blend to an oriental type.

Contraindications: May cause irritation on sensitive skin.

GRAPEFRUIT   Latin name: *Citrus paradisi*

Family species: *Rutaceae*

Purchasing guide: **Color:** Yellow to pale green; **Viscosity:** Watery; **Aroma:** Warm, sweet, fresh citrus. *A citrus oil should be used within six months of purchase.*

Countries of origin: USA, South Africa, Israel, Brazil

Description: Small tree with dark, evergreen leaves and large, creamy-white flowers and large, yellow fruits.

Part used: Fresh peel

Extraction method: Cold-pressed

Yield: 0.5–1%

Most valuable uses: Muscle fatigue, stiffness, cellulite, headaches, acne, mental exhaustion, hangovers, fluid retention, antiseptic, disinfectant, detoxification

Therapeutic properties: Tonic, digestive, depurative, antiseptic, anti-infectious, restorative

Main chemical components: D Limonene, gamma Terpinene, Nootketone, Cadinene, Neral, Citronellal

Blends well with: Ginger, juniper, cypress, clary sage, clove, palmarosa, ylang ylang, mandarin, lavender, geranium, rosemary, thyme linalol, peppermint, eucalyptus (all), fennel, black pepper, frankincense, patchouli

Interesting facts: The plant was introduced into the West Indies from China by a Captain Shaddock and the fruit was thereafter known as "Shaddock fruit." In 1809 the seeds traveled with Spanish settlers to the United States, but grapefruit was not grown here commercially until 1880. In many parts of the world the waste products of this and other citrus fruits are ground and used as animal fodder.

Contraindications: None known.

HELICHRYSUM (Italian Everlasting)

Latin names: *Helichrysum augustifolium, H italicum, H orientale*

Family species: *Asteraceae (Compositae)*

Purchasing guide: **Color:** Pale yellow; **Viscosity:** Watery; **Aroma:** Powerful, fruity, fresh, straw-like

Countries of origin: France, Corsica, Hungary

Description: Evergreen herb growing up to 20 inches tall, with long stems, off which grow many thin, needle-like, velvety leaflets. At the top of each stem is a clump of about 30 small flower-heads which are covered in bright yellow scales.

Part used: Yellow flowering-head clusters

Extraction method: Steam distillation

Yield: 0.01–0.09%

Most valuable uses: Pain relief, bruising, general tonic, coughs, bronchial congestion, scarring, circulatory disorders, rheumatism, arthritis

Therapeutic properties: Anti-spasmodic, analgesic, cicatrisive, expectorant, anticoagulant, hepatic, cholagogue, anti-inflammatory, stimulant

Main chemical components: Neryl Acetate, Nerol, Geraniol, Linalol

Blends well with: Bergamot, black pepper, cedarwood, chamomile german, clary sage, cypress, frankincense, geranium, grapefruit, juniper, lavender, lemon, mandarin, naiouli, oregano, palmarosa, ravensara, pine, rosemary, sage, tea tree, thyme linalol, rose maroc, rose otto, ylang ylang, vetiver, eucalyptus citriodora

Interesting facts: Flowers are used in dry-flower arrangements. There are about 500 species of helichrysum, of which only a few produce essential oil for distillation. Romans used helichrysum to repel moths from their houses. Listed in Greco-Roman, and Medieval European texts as a medicinal herb. Used throughout Europe as a strewing-herb — a plant material that can be crushed underfoot to create a pleasant aroma and/or deter bugs.

Contraindications: Not to be used on children under 12. Not to be used during pregnancy. Use in moderation.

HYACINTH   Latin name: *Hyacinthus orientalis*

Family species: *Liliaceae*

Purchasing guide: **Color:** Brownish-green; **Viscosity:** Viscous; **Aroma:** Powerful, hypnotic, green, deep, soft, floral. *Only a small amount is used in a blend, diluted, as it is very strong. Synthetics are sometimes sold as naturals.*

Countries of origin: Holland, France, Egypt

Description: Perennial herbaceous bulbous plant, with thin, slender, light to dark green leaves and large flower heads with bell-shaped flowers, often pink but other colors are used, such as blue and white.

Part used: Flowers

Extraction method: Solvent extraction then alcohol extraction which produces an absolute

Yield: 0.01–0.02%

Most valuable uses: For use in aroma-psychology, emotional crisis, sedative, stress, tension, calming, mental tiredness, sorrow, feelings of distress and neglect.

Therapeutic properties: Hypnotic, sedative, antidepressant, antiseptic

Main chemical components: Benzyl Alcohol, troxo cinnamly alcohol, Benzaldehyde, Phenylethyl-alcohol

Blends well with: Rose maroc, rose otto, lemon, bergamot, grapefruit, litsea cubeba, neroli, ylang ylang, frankincense, orange, cypress, sandalwood, petitgrain, geranium

Interesting facts: Named by Linnaeus after Hyacinthus, a Spartan youth beloved by Apollo and Zephyrus. The ancient Greeks used the fragrance for emotional problems. The bulbs are often grown in water to show the long white root system to school children. When grown in the house the fragrance can fill a room when left overnight.

Contraindications: None known.

JASMINE	Latin names: *Jasminum grandiflorum, J officinale, J sambac*

Family species: *Oleaceae*

Purchasing guide: Color: Deep, orangish-brown; **Viscosity:** viscous; **Aroma:** Sweet rich floral, honey-like

Countries of origin: France, India, Morocco, Egypt, Algeria, China

Description: Fragile climbing bush that grows up to 33 feet high, with dark green leaves and small, white, star-shaped flowers, which grow well on young shoots. (*J Odoratissimum* and some Chinese varieties, and those found in Nepal, produce yellow flowers).

Part used: flowers

Extraction method: The aromatic molecules are known as an "absolute." This is extracted from "concretes" or "pomades," themselves produced by enfleurage of the flowers, or by CO_2 extraction with natural solvents.

Yield: 1,000 lbs of flowers yields approximately one pound of liquid concrete, which yields 0.2% of aromatic molecules. Fifty per cent of this could yield jasmin absolute.

Most valuable uses: Aphrodisiac, fertility, nervous tension, stress-related conditions, depression, antiseptic, skin care

Therapeutic properties: Antidepressant, stimulant, aphrodisiac, antiseptic, anti-spasmodic, cicatrisive, sedative

Main chemical components: Benzyl Acetate, Linalol, Linalyl Acetate, Benzyl Alcohol, Jasmone, Methyl-jasmonate, Indole

Blends well with: Rose maroc, rose otto, neroli, sandalwood, palmarosa, geranium, lemon, clove, grapefruit, clary sage, bergamot, mandarin, orange, patchouli, petitgrain, ylang ylang, coriander, benzoin, bay, ginger

Interesting facts: Name derived from the Persian *yasmin.* Flowers must be picked before the sun rises. An experienced picker can pick between 10,000–15,000 blossoms per day. More than 200 species of jasmine worldwide. Indians string the flowers together as garlands for honored guests. In China, the flowers are used to fragrance tea. Used medicinally in China, India, and Arabia. Very important oil to the perfume industry.

Contraindications: None known.

JUNIPER   Latin name: *Juniperus communis*

Family species: *Cupressaceae*

Purchasing guide: **Color:** Colorless to pale yellow; **Viscosity:** Watery; **Aroma:** Fresh, fruity, woody, gin-type

Countries of origin: Italy, France, Hungary, Spain, Canada

Description: Shrubby looking tree can grow to over 30 ft. Sometimes has a divided trunk with a brownish gray wood. The leaves are pointed like needles, a feathery bluish-green, arranged in groups of three. There are male and female trees; only the female tree produces a bluish gray ball type fruit (sometimes called a berry).

Part used: Dried, crushed, or slightly dried ripe fruit

Extraction method: Steam distillation

Yield: 0.2%–2%

Most valuable uses: Fluid retention, rheumatism, ulcers, arthritis, acne, eczema, obesity, gout, mental exhaustion, infections, nervous tension, toxicity, overindulgence of food, cystitis, sciatica, hay fever, premenstrual bloating

Therapeutic properties: Antiseptic, diuretic, expectorant, emmenagogue, anti-parasitic, tonic, depurative

Main chemical components: Alpha Pinene, Sabinene, Myrcene, Camphene, Terpineol

Blends well with: Rosemary, geranium, lavender, lemon, grapefruit, sandalwood, cypress, clary sage, pine, frankincense, vetiver, cedarwood, sage, mandarin, eucalyptus (all), bergamot, fennel, rose otto

Interesting facts: The berries were well known in Egypt, ancient China, and Tibet, where they were used as medicines and for purifying. During the plagues of the Middle Ages in Europe, juniper was used as a defense against such disease as smallpox. Juniper berries are still used in the manufacture of gin. A different essence is obtained from the branches — known as cade oil, it is used in veterinary care.

Contraindications: Not to be used during pregnancy. Not to be used on children under 12 years. Not to be used by those with kidney problems.

LAVENDER	**Latin names:** *Lavendula Angustifolia, L officinalis, L vera, L fragrans*

Family species: *Labiatae (Lamiaceae)*

Purchasing guide: Color: Clear; **Viscosity:** Watery; **Aroma:** Fresh, herbaceous, floral

Countries of origin: France, China, England, Tasmania, Bulgaria, Russia, Croatia

Description: A herbaceous bushy plant reaching a height of four feet. A woody plant with spike-shaped leaves of light greyish green. They have a downy look, the flowers appearing in various shades of mauve to violet-lavender, which are tightly packed around a singular stem.

Part used: Flowering tops

Extraction method: Steam distillation

Yield: 1.4–1.6%

Most valuable uses: Cuts, grazes, burns, rheumatism, chilblains, dermatitis, eczema, sunburn, insect bites, headaches, migraine, insomnia, infections, arthritis, anxiety, tension, panic, hysteria, fatigue, inflammatory conditions, rashes, nervous conditions, dysmenorrhoea, spasms. Can be used safely on children.

Therapeutic properties: Antiseptic, analgesic, cytophylactic, anti-spasmodic, tonic, cicatrisive, anti-inflammatory, emmenagogue, anti-venomous, anti-toxic, anti-parasitic, antitussive, diuretic, restorative, decongestant, antidepressant, calmative, sedative, antibiotic, anti-infectious

Main chemical components: Linalyl Acetate, Linalool, Geraniol, Borneol, Isoborneol, Cineol-1,8

Blends well with: Chamomile roman, chamomile german, lemon, geranium, eucalyptus (all), thyme linalol, rosemary, tea tree, peppermint, grapefruit, clary sage, palmarosa, mandarin, juniper, cypress, pine, black pepper, marjoram, cedarwood, bergamot, lemongrass, ravensara

Interesting facts: The name is derived from the Roman word *lavera*, "to wash," as the Romans used the flowers in their baths. It has been cultivated since ancient times. In modern times, once planted, it will yield oil for up to ten years, depending upon the species. Lavender is used to ward off insects, in closets, etc., and used in perfumery and cooking. It is said to be an antidote against the bites of funnel web spider, black widow, and certain snakes such as vipers and adders.

Contraindications: None known.

LEMON   Latin name: *Citrus limonum*

Family species: *Rutaceae*

Purchasing guide: Color: Pale yellow with greenish tint; **Viscosity:** Watery; **Aroma:** Light, clean, fresh, citrus. *Shelf life of only 8–10 months.*

Countries of origin: Brazil, USA, Argentina, Italy, Israel

Description: Tree growing up to 16 feet, with dark green leaves and branches which bear small "spines" (from which an essential oil of lemon-petitgrain is derived). The highly perfumed, white flowers are always in bloom. Produces yellow fruits.

Part used: Fresh fruit peel

Extraction method: Cold expression

Yield: 0.6–0.8%

Most valuable uses: General tonic, infections, detoxification, general fatigue, obesity, acne, physical exhaustion, digestion, depression, rheumatism, colds and flu, skin care

Therapeutic properties: Antibiotic, sedative, carminative, diuretic, haemostatic, astringent, digestive, immunostimulant, antidepressant, stimulant, antiseptic, febrifuge, calmative, antispasmodic, antisclerotic, depuratve, vermifuge, cicatrisive

Main chemical components: D Limonene, Citral, gamma Terpinene, Phellandrene, Citronellal, Citroptene

Blends well with: All other essential oils

Interesting facts: The name comes from the Persian or Arabic, *limun*, which in turn may derive from the Indian Sanskrit — the lemon tree was thought to have originally come from northeast India. Thought be brought to Europe from Arabia. The tree was introduced into California in 1887. The oil is effective in removing ink stains and polishing metal, and as a solvent for computers. The juice is a source of citric acid. For many years the British Navy was required to provide sailors with one ounce daily, to alleviate scurvy and other vitamin-deficiency problems. The essential oil is full of vitamins and minerals. Used diffused in the atmosphere in banks and other commercial buildings in Japan to reduce worker-error.

Contraindications: Do not apply neat to the skin. Do not apply to the skin before exposure to the sun.

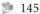

LEMONGRASS　　　Latin name: *Cymbopogon flexuosus*

Family species: *Graminacea*

Purchasing guide: Color: Dark yellow; **Viscosity:** Watery; **Aroma:** Lemony, straw-like, green

Countries of origin: India, Sri Lanka, Madagascar, Guatemala, Nepal

Description: Perennial grass growing to 4 feet, with long, thin leaves which bend and fall toward the ground in a untidy, disheveled manner.

Part used: Leaves

Extraction method: Steam distillation of fresh or partly dried leaves

Yield: 1.8–2.2%

Most valuable uses: Infections, acne, general tonic, digestion, diuretic, nervous conditions, cellulite, skin care

Therapeutic properties: Astringent, tonic, calmative, antiseptic, anti-infectious, diuretic, digestive, anti-parasitic, depurative, nervine

Main chemical components: Citral, n-decylic aldehyde, Dipentene, Farucsol, Neral, Citronellal, Geranial

Blends well with: Basil, bergamot, black pepper, cedarwood, clary sage, coriander, cypress, fennel, geranium, ginger, grapefruit, lavender, lemon, marjoram, orange, patchouli, palmarosa, rosemary, tea tree, thyme linalol, vetiver, ylang ylang

Interesting facts: Used as an insect deterrent. Used in Ayurvedic medicine (traditional Indian). An important component of Indian and other Asian cooking. The essential oil is used in perfumery and citrus-type soaps.

Contraindications: None known.

LINDEN BLOSSOM	Latin names: *Tilia cordata, T europoea, T platyphyllos*

Family species: *Tiliaceae*

Purchasing guide: Color: Greenish; **Viscosity:** Viscous; **Aroma:** Light, floral, sweet

Country of origin: France

Description: Deciduous tree growing to 100 feet high with wide, heart-shaped leaves with a whitish down on the underside, particularly on the veins. The small, extremely fragrant white flowers grow in drooping clusters on long stalks. Some trees are thought to be over 1,000 years old.

Part used: Flowers

Extraction method: The aromatic molecules are known as an "absolute". This is extracted from "concretes" or "pomades", themselves produced by enflourage of the flowers, or by CO_2 extraction with natural solvents.

Yield: 0.05%

Most valuable uses: Used in aroma-psychology, nervous tension, insomnia, constant thinking, anxiety, emotional crisis, sadness, hysteria

Therapeutic properties: Anti-spasmodic, emollient, sedative, diuretic, antidepressant, astringent, nervine, tonic, calmative, antiseptic

Main chemical components: Farnesol

Blends well with: Frankincense, geranium, jasmine, rose maroc, rose otto, mandarin, neroli, petitgrain, sandalwood, ylang ylang, black pepper, clove

Interesting facts: Often called "lime tree" although no limes grow from it. The insect-repellent wood is used in organ and piano manufacture, as wood carving material, and artist's charcoal. The leaves have been used to adulterate tobacco. The flowers are used extensively in European herbal medicine and many households collect the flowers to make a medicinal tea. The flowers also attract bees which make an excellent honey.

Contraindications: None known.

LITSEA CUBEBA (May-Chang Oil)
Latin name: *Litsea citrata*

Family species: *Lauraceae*

Purchasing guide: **Color:** Pale yellow to yellow; **Viscosity:** Watery; **Aroma:** Sweet, smoky, lemony

Countries of origin: China, Java

Description: Shrub-like tree growing up to 30 feet, belonging to the laurel family, the bright green lance-shaped leaves have slender branches bearing fluffy white flowers and small, green, round green fruits, about the size of a peppercorn.

Part used: Ripe fruit

Extraction method: Steam distillation

Yield: 2%

Most valuable uses: Nervousness, general tonic, relaxing, skin care, acne, indigestion, depression, anxiety, stress, poor appetite, anorexia, cleansing, tissue toning, cellulite

Therapeutic properties: Calmative, anti-infectious, antibiotic, stimulant, vulnerary, antiseptic, stomachic, antidepressant

Main chemical components: Citral, Neral, Geranial, Linalool

Blends well with: Bay, basil, benzoin, black pepper, cardamom, cedarwood, chamomile roman, clary sage, coriander, cypress, eucalyptus citriodora, eucalyptus radiata, frankincense, geranium, ginger, grapefruit, juniper, marjoram, orange, patchouli, palmarosa, petitgrain, rosemary, sandalwood, tea tree, thyme linalol, vetiver, ylang ylang

Interesting facts: The name *cubeba* is given to this plant because the small round fruits resemble those on the climbing shrub *piper cubeba*, a native plant of Java. The fruit of the tree is also made into a hot flavoring for meat known as sambal; while the flowers are used as flavoring for tea. The oil is used widely in citrus-type perfumes.

Contraindications: None known.

MANDARIN	Latin name: *Citrus madurensis, C nobilis, C reticulara*

Family species: *Rutaceae*

Purchasing guide: Color: Yellow gold; **Viscosity:** Watery; **Aroma:** Sweet, light, floral, fruity citrus

Countries of origin: USA, Brazil, Italy, Algeria, Tunisia, Spain, Argentina, China

Description: Small evergreen tree with creamy-white scented flowers, producing small, flattened-round, loose skinned, orange fruits.

Part used: Rind of the fruit

Extraction method: Cold expression

Yield: 0.7–0.8%

Most valuable uses: Convalescence, digestive problems, exhaustion, nervous tension, irritability, cellulite, constipation, skin care

Therapeutic properties: Tonic, stomachic, digestive, calmative, anti-spasmodic, antiseptic

Main chemical components: D Limonene, gamma Terpinene, Geraniol, Citral, Citronellal

Blends well with: Lemon, grapefruit, geranium, clove, palmarosa, clary sage, ylang ylang, juniper, jasmine, rose maroc, rose otto, neroli, basil, black pepper, chamomile roman, frankincense, myrrh, patchouli, petitgrain, sandalwood, cinnamon

Interesting facts: The name comes from the mandarins of Cochin China, where it originates, and to whom the fruit was offered as a gift. Not to be confused with tangerine.

Contraindications: Do not use on the skin before exposure to the sun.

MANUKA   Latin name: *Leptospermum scoparium*

Family species: *Myrtaceae*

Purchasing guide: Color: Yellow; **Viscosity:** Watery; **Aroma:** Sweet, camphorous, shrubby

Country of origin: New Zealand

Description: Narrow shrub or small tree with deep red wood, and small, dark, pointed, concave leaves with small (2 cm) flowers, either pink or red.

Part used: Leaves and end-branches

Extraction method: Steam distillation

Yield: 1.5–2%

Most valuable uses: Athlete's foot, ringworm, thrush, skin infections, colds, flu, sore throats, rheumatism, muscular pain, urinary infections, intestinal infections, burns, wounds

Therapeutic properties: Antibiotic, anti-fungal, antiseptic, anti-infectious, analgesic, vulnerary

Main chemical components: Beta-caryphyllen, Geraniol, Geranial, Linalol, Alpha-pinene, Geranuylacetate

Blends well with: Basil, bergamot, black pepper, chamomile roman, chamomile german, clary sage, cypress, eucalyptus (all), geranium, grapefruit, lavender, lemon, marjoram, orange, patchouli, peppermint, petitgrain, pine, ravensara, rosemary, sage, sandalwood, tea tree, thyme linalol, thyme red, litsea cubeba, yuzu

Interesting facts: All parts of this plant have been used by the Maori people as an important part of their natural medicine. When Captain Cook and his men arrived in New Zealand they came across this bush and used it for making tea. Cook wrote, "it has a very agreeable bitter taste and flavor when (the leaves) are recent but loses some of both when they are dried." But, as they discovered, if made too strong, the tea can make a person vomit. Manuka was the original "tea tree." Also grows in Australia.

Contraindications: None known.

| **MARJORAM** (sweet) | **Latin name:** *Origanum marjorana (Marjorana hortensis)* |

Family species: *Labiatae*

Purchasing guide: **Color:** Colorless to pale yellow/amber; **Viscosity:** Medium; **Aroma:** Warm, spicy, herbaceous. *Often confused with thyme and oregano essential oils.*

Countries of origin: Spain, France, Tunisia, Morocco, Egypt, Bulgaria, Hungary, Germany

Description: Perennial herb growing to over one foot high, with a downy stem and small, silver-green downy leaves with tiny, pinkish-white flowers.

Part used: Fresh and dried leaves and flowering tops

Extraction method: Steam distillation

Yield: 0.5–3%

Most valuable uses: Muscle relaxant, muscular stiffness, bronchitis, colds, head congestion, constipation, cleansing, circulation, feeling cold, menstrual problems, tension, anxiety, general debility, sore throats

Therapeutic properties: Analgesic, anti-spasmodic, vasodilator, calmative, expectorant, anti-aphrodisiac, sedative, vagotonic, digestive, vulnery, antitussive, antiseptic, antibiotic, anti-infectious, diuretic, emmenagogue

Main chemical components: Terpinene-4-ol, alpha Terpineol, alpha Terpinene, Sabinene, Para-cymeme

Blends well with: Basil, bergamot, black pepper, chamomile roman, chamomile german, cedarwood, clary sage, cypress, eucalyptus citriodora, eucalyptus radiata, fennel, juniper, lavender, lemon, orange, peppermint, pine, rosemary, tea tree, thyme linalol

Interesting facts: Grown as a potted herb by the ancient Egyptians. Used in unguents and perfumes since known records. Greek women used an oil infused with marjoram on their heads, as a relaxant. Plant used in the 16th century Europe, strewn on the floors of rooms. Traditionally, it is said that if you place a bunch of marjoram near milk it will not go sour.

Contraindications: None known.

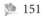

MELISSA Latin name: *Melissa officinalis*

Family species: *Labiatae (Lamiaceae)*

Purchasing guide: Color: Pale yellow; **Viscosity:** Watery; **Aroma:** Citrus, light, fresh

Because Melissa's yield is extremely low, this oil is very expensive. Worldwide, the amount reported sold far exceeds the amount produced, indicating that this oil is being adulterated. A trustworthy supplier is essential.

Countries of origin: France, Ireland

Description: Perennial herb, growing to three feet, very bushy, which self-propagates extremely well. The small, serrated leaves are lemon-scented. The plant produces small, pinkish-white flowers, which grow off the stem, at the base of the leaves.

Part used: Flowering tops, leaves and stems

Extraction method: Steam distillation of fresh parts

Yield: 0.01–0.02%

Most valuable uses: Calming, stomach cramps, nausea, palpitations, stress, depression, headache, intellectual fatigue, menstrual pain, general tonic, herpes, candida

Therapeutic properties: Antiseptic, antibiotic, anti-viral, sedative, calmative, antidepressant, stimulant, stomachic

Main chemical components: Neral, Geranial, Methyl heptenone, Citronellai, Citral, Linalol, Copaene, Germacrene

Blends well with: Chamomile roman, rose maroc, rose otto, neroli, petitgrain, geranium, frankincense. *Most often used alone.*

Interesting facts: Also known as lemon balm. Melissa was used by Paracelsus, who said it was a powerful reviver. Very attractive to bees. The herb is used in salads, egg dishes, vinegar and tea.

Contraindications: None known.

MYRRH	Latin name: *Commiphora myrrha*

Family species: *Burseraceae*

Purchasing guide: Color: Reddish-brownish-orange; **Viscosity:** Viscous; **Aroma:** Warm, slightly musty, earthy

Countries of origin: Somalia, Ethiopia, Sudan, southern Arabia

Description: Very thorny, short, sturdy tree, growing to nine feet, with light bark, and knotted branches that stand at right-angles to the trunk. Very few, small oval leaves, and small white flowers. Natural fissures or deliberate wounds made to the bark produce a pale yellow liquid which hardens to a reddish-brown color, the mass being about the size of a walnut although, being brittle, it can easily be reduced in size. This is the oleo-resin-gum.

Part used: Oleoresin-gum

Extraction method: Steam distillation of the oleoresin-gum

Yield: 3–5%

Most valuable uses: Coughs, catarrh, bronchitis, ulcerations, mouth ulcers, colds, wounds, infections, feeling cold, eczema, ringworm, sores, chapped skin, gum infections, skin care

Therapeutic properties: Pectoral, antiseptic, anti-spasmodic, cicatrisive, balsamic, expectorant, anti-fungal, astringent, vulnerary

Main chemical components: Mono & Sesquiterpenes, commiphoric acid

Blends well with: Frankincense, sandalwood, cypress, juniper, geranium, lavender, lemon, palmarosa, tea tree, eucalyptus citriodora, eucalyptus radiata, rosemary, chamomile roman, bergamot, grapefruit, patchouli, pine, vetiver, ylang ylang

Interesting facts: Used for over 4,000 years. The ancient Egyptians used it in their *Kyphi* incense and in embalming. Also included in the popular ancient Greek perfume, *megaleion*. Thought to have been one of the materials used by the Queen of Sheba in her seduction of King Solomon. The resin is flammable and burns easily. One of the gifts given to baby Jesus on his birth.

Contraindications: Not to be used during pregnancy.

NEROLI	Latin name: *Citrus aurantium,* *C brigaradia, C vulgaris*

Family species: *Rutacea*

Purchasing guide: **Color:** Pale yellow; **Viscosity:** Watery; **Aroma:** Highly radiant, sweet, floral. *An absolute is also made with fresh flowers. Sometimes adult-erated with petitgrain.*

Countries of origin: Italy (Calabria), Tunisia, Morocco Algeria, France

Description: Made from the small, white, waxy flowers of the bitter-orange tree which grows between 18–30 feet high. A hybrid is cultivated in Florida.

Part used: Fresh flowers, hand picked just before they open

Extraction method: Steam distillation

Yield: 0.8–1%

Most valuable uses: Nervousness, calming, insomnia, scar tissue, skin care, depression, tension, PMS, palpitations, convalescence, fear, shock, stretch marks, intestinal spasm

Therapeutic properties: Sedative, antidepressant, anti-infectious, antibiotic, tonic, cytophylactic, calmative, cicatrisive, aphrodisiac

Main chemical components: Pinenes, Limonene, Linalyl Acetate, Linalol, Nerolidol, Nerol, Geraniol, Citral

Blends well with: Geranium, camomile roman, coriander, benzoin, clary sage, frankincense, mandarin, orange, petit-grain, jasmine, rose maroc, rose otto, ylang ylang, yuzu, lemon, grapefruit, mandarin, lavender, palmarosa, ginger, sandalwood, juniper

Interesting facts: The essential oil is also known as "orange blossom." It takes 1,000 lbs. of blossoms to make one lb. of oil. Named after the Prince of Nerola, Flavio Orsini of 16th century Italy, who went to great lengths to ensure a supply for his wife, Anna-Maria de la Tremoille, who loved the fragrance and made it fashionable. Very often associated with marriage purity. Traditionally, brides wore the flowers in their hair. An ingredient in eau de colognes.

Contraindications: None known.

| ORANGE | Latin name: *Citrus aurantium, C sinensis, C brigarade* |

Family species: *Rutacea*

Purchasing guide: **Color:** Yellow to orange; **Viscosity:** Watery; **Aroma:** Fresh, fruity, tangy, sweet *"Bitter orange" essential oil is made from* Citrus aurantium *while "sweet orange" is derived from* Citrus sinensis. *Shelf-life is approximately six months.*

Countries of origin: China, Israel, Morocco, Tunisia, Algeria, Italy, France, USA

Description: Small tree with dark green leaves and white flowers, and bright orange round fruit with roughish skin.

Part used: Orange peel

Extraction method: Cold-pressed

Yield: 0.3–0.5%

Most valuable uses: Diuretic, constipation, helps eliminate toxins, overindulgence, skin care, antiseptic, nervous anxiety, disinfectant, general body tonic

Therapeutic properties: Calmative, anticoagulant, sedative, stomachic, cholagogue, diuretic, tonic, anti-spasmodic, antiseptic, antibiotic, depurative

Main chemical components: D Limonene, n-decylic aldehyde, Linalool, Terpineol, B-carotin

Blends well with: Bay, benzoin, bergamot, black pepper, cinnamon, clove, coriander, eucalyptus citriodora, frankincense, geranium, ginger, grapefruit, juniper, lemon, litsea cubeba, marjoram, neroli, patchouli, petitgrain, sandalwood, vetiver, jasmine, ylang ylang, rose maroc, rose otto

Interesting facts: Contains vitamins, minerals, and enzymes. Originated in China. The oil is used for flavoring food, drink and confectionery. Also used in many Curacao type liqueurs and for flavoring cigarette paper. The orange tree was taken to the West coast of America by Franciscan monks, who began the cultivation of it there. Ignites at 75° Fahrenheit (23° Centigrade). Protects against insect damage when added to furniture polish.

Contraindications: As with all citrus essential oils, should not be applied to the skin before exposure to strong sunlight.

OREGANO   **Latin name:** *Origanum vulgare*

Family species: *Labiatae (Labiaceae)*

Purchasing guide: **Color:** Pale yellow; **Viscosity:** Medium to watery; **Aroma:** Powerful, herbaceous, spicy camphor-like.

Countries of origin: Morocco, Spain, France, USA, Italy

Description: Perennial densely branched herb growing to 20 inches, with oval leaves, producing a profusion of pink flowers clustered in heads at the tops of the branches.

Part used: Dried, flowering tops

Extraction method: Steam distillation

Yield: 1–3%

Most valuable uses: Respiratory infection, bronchitis, rheumatism, arthritis, general debility, muscular pain, infections, colds, flu

Therapeutic properties: Anti-infectious, antibiotic, anti-viral, antiseptic, stimulant, anti-aphrodisiac, emmenagogue, anti-parasitic, expectorant, rubefacient

Main chemical components: Carvacrol, Thymol, Terpinene, Cymene, Menthene

Blends well with: Lavender, bay, bergamot, chamomile roman, cypress, eucalyptus (all), lemon, litsea cubeba, orange, petitgrain, rosemary, tea tree, thyme linalol, thyme red

Interesting facts: Plant is favored by bees. The herb is used extensively in Mediterranean cooking. The essential oil is used in dental preparations.

Contraindications: Not to be used during pregnancy. Not to be used on children under 18. Can cause skin irritation, so best used in a diffuser. Do not use in baths.

ORMENIS FLOWER (Chamomile Maroc) — Latin name: *Ormenis multicaulis*

Family species: *Asteraceae (Compositae)*

Purchasing guide: **Color:** Pale to darkish yellow; **Viscosity:** Watery; **Aroma:** Balsamic, herby, sweet

Country of origin: Morocco

Description: Plant growing to three feet high, with tubular yellow and white flowers and hairy leaves.

Part used: Flowering tops

Extraction method: Steam distillation

Yield: 1.5–2%

Most valuable uses: Colitis, dermatitis, nervousness, tension, stress, general tonic, insomnia, irritability, menstrual problems, menopause, rheumatism, anxiety, skin care

Therapeutic properties: Anti-infectious, antibiotic, tonic, anti-parasitic, emmenagogue, anti-spasmodic, sedative, calmative, antiseptic

Main chemical components: Santolina Alcohol, a-terpineol, camphore, 1,8 cineol, a-pinene, yomogi alcohol

Blends well with: Bay, benzoin, bergamot, black pepper, cardadom, chamomile roman, clary sage, coriander, frankincense, geranium, grapefruit, jasmine, lavender, lemon, lemongrass, mandarin, marjoram, orange, patchouli, petitgrain, rose maroc, sandalwood, ylang ylang, yuzu

Interesting facts: Often sold as "chamomile" and spoken of as a chamomile. Although the plant is similar in appearance the essential oil is distinct from true chamomiles — not having the same therapeutic or chemical characteristics — and should not be confused with them. Sometimes known as "chamomile mixta." The flowers are made into teas around the Meditteranean area and North Africa. The essential oil is used in perfumery. It is also sometimes used to adulterate essential oil of cistus.

Contraindications: None known.

PALMAROSA	**Latin name:** *Cymbopogon martini Stapf., subspecies motia*

Family species: *Graminaceae*

Purchasing guide: **Color:** Pale yellow to olive; **Viscosity:** Medium to watery; **Aroma:** Sweet, rosy, floral, lemony. *The subspecies* motia, *meaning "precious," is the true palmarosa oil; the subspecies* sofia, *meaning "mediocre," is the source of gingergrass oil.*

Countries of origin: Nepal, India, Brazil, Central America

Description: A green and straw-colored grass with long stems ending in tufts, which produce small yellow flowers.

Part used: Fresh or dried grass, harvested before it flowers

Extraction method: Steam distillation

Yield: 1–1.5%

Most valuable uses: Physical exhaustion, stress-related problems, convalescence, acne, scarring, tissue regeneration, skin care, nervousness, anorexia, intestinal infections, athlete's foot and other fungal infections, eczema, general fatigue, uterine tonic, vaginal infections

Therapeutic properties: Antibiotic, anti-fungal, anti-viral, tonic, anti-infectious, antiseptic, vermifuge, cytophylactic, digestive, emollient, nervine, cicatrisive, stimulant

Main chemical components: Geraniol, Geranyl acetate, Linalool, alpha humulene, beta caryophyllene

Blends well with: Geranium, grapefruit, clary sage, ginger, ylang-ylang, sandalwood, mandarin, juniper, lemon, clove, rosemary, chamomile roman, rose maroc, rose otto, bay, benzoin, bergamot, coriander, frankincense, lemongrass, lemon, orange, petitgrain, patchouli, clove

Interesting facts: Used to be called "Turkish geranium oil" or "East Indian geranium oil." Because the high geraniol content makes it smell rose-like, palmarosa is often used to adulterate rose essential oil. It is shaken with gum arabic solution and left in the sun — a process which makes it lighter in color, thus more like rose oil.

Contraindications: None known.

PATCHOULI — Latin name: *Pogostemon Cablin*

Family species: *Labiacae (Labiata)*

Purchasing guide: **Color:** Reddish-brown; **Viscosity:** Viscous; **Aroma:** Earthy, sweet, herbaceous, smoky, *Sometimes adulterated with cubeb or Cedar wood oils.*

Countries of origin: Indonesia, Malaysia, Philippines, Madagascar, China, India

Description: Large, hairy herbaceous perennial bush growing to about three feet high, bearing white flowers with a purple hue.

Part used: Non-flower leaves

Extraction method: Steam distillation of sun-dried, slightly fermented leaves

Yield: 2–3%

Most valuable uses: Fungal infections, bacterial infections, constipation, uterine tonic, dandruff, insect repellent, insect bites, stress-related emotional disorders, substance addictions, dermatitis, athlete's foot, ringworm, parasites, helps eliminate toxins

Therapeutic properties: Tonic, cytophylactic, anti-infectious, antiseptic, decongestant, antibiotic, anti-fungal, anti-depressant, anti-toxic, aphrodisiac, astringent, calmative, nervine

Main chemical components: Patchouli Alcohol, Pogostol, Patchoulene, Patchoulenol, Sesquiterpene

Blends well with: Bergamot, black pepper, chamomile german, cedarwood, clary sage, frankincense, clove, geranium, grapefruit, jasmine, myrrh, rose maroc, mandarin, neroli, orange, sandalwood, vetiver, ylang ylang, coriander, ginger, lemongrass, cinnamon, litsea cubeba, yuzu

Interesting facts: Possibly originated in Malaysia although the word apparently comes from the south Indian Tamil language, *patch*, meaning "green," and *ilai* meaning "leaf." As well as for perfume and medicine, patchouli is used for scenting carpets, shawls and woven materials, and for perfuming ink.

Contraindications: None known.

PEPPERMINT   Latin name: *Mentha piperita*

Family species: *Lamiaceae (Labiatae)*

Purchasing guide: Color: Clear to pale yellow; **Viscosity:** Watery; **Aroma:** Camphorous, minty fresh. *Important to buy from a good source as sometimes not enough attention is given to the cropping, so weeds are sometimes distilled with the peppermint plant. Other species such as* Menta Arvensis (Cornmint) *are also used in aromatherapy.*

Countries of Origin: USA, England, France, Italy, Russia, China

Description: Perennial plant growing to about two feet high, with small leaves and pinkish-mauve flowers arranged in a long, conical shape.

Part used: Whole plant above ground, just before flowering

Extraction method: Steam distillation of fresh or partially dried plant

Yield: 0.1–1.0%

Most valuable uses: Headaches, nausea, fatigue, apathy, coughs, digestive problems, bowel disorders, flatulence, muscular pain, sinus congestion, shock, faintness, travel sickness, mouth or gum infections, mental tiredness, poor circulation

Therapeutic properties: Antiseptic, antibiotic, anti-infectious, carminative, stomachic, anti-spasmodic, depurative, stimulant, tonic, emmenagogue, anti-parasitic, vermifuge, expectorant, analgesic, digestive, decongestant

Main chemical components: Menthol, Menthone, iso Menthone, Menthofuran, Menthol ester

Blends well with: Basil, pine, lemon, geranium, rosemary, tea tree, lavender, eucalyptus (all), grapefruit, juniper, cypress, black pepper, niaouli, ravensara

Interesting facts: According to Greek mythology the genus *Mentha* takes its name from the nymph Minthe who was seduced by Pluto and turned into a plant by his jealous wife, who trod Mintha into the ground. Pluto, however, turned her into a herb, knowing Minthe would then be appreciated by people for years to come. Cultivation began in the USA in 1855 in Indiana, New York, and Ohio.

Contraindications: Could cause irritation if applied neat to the skin. Do not use in baths. Not to be used in pregnancy or on children under seven years.

PETITGRAIN	Latin name: *Citrus aurantium, ss C amara, C brigaradier*

Family species: *Rutacea*

Purchasing guide: **Color:** Pale yellow; **Viscosity:** Watery; **Aroma:** Warm, sharp, woody, floral

Countries of origin: France, Italy, Tunisia, Morocco, USA, Paraguay, Brazil

Description: Made from the dark green, glossy leaves and small leaf-bearing twigs of the orange tree, and the small, seed-like, green fruit buds which are left after the flowers have fallen. In Paraguay and in Brazil the trees grow wild as well as being cultivated.

Part used: Fresh leaves and small twigs, and in very high quality oil, also the small, unripe green fruit

Extraction method: Steam distillation

Yield: 0.5–1%

Most valuable uses: Calming, nervous conditions, acne, insomnia, depression, general debility, anxiety, stress-related conditions, indigestion, skin care

Therapeutic properties: Anti-spasmodic, antidepressant, stimulant, tonic, calmative, anti-infectious, antiseptic, nervine

Main chemical components: Linalyl Acetate, Linalol, Geranyl acetate, Nerol, Terpineol, Nerolidol

Blends well with: Rosemary, clary sage, basil, bergamot, benzoin, clove, cedarwood, cypress, eucalyptus citriodora, frankincense, geranium, jasmine, juniper, lavender, lemon, mandarin, marjoram, neroli, orange, palmarosa, patchouli, rose maroc, rose otto, sandalwood, ylang ylang, yuzu

Interesting facts: The name "petitgrain" is derived from the word for little fruits or little grains. Used in classic eau de colognes. In 1694 it was distilled from the small unripe fruits called orangettes, which are seeds or kernels. The trees are pruned in June which gives the material for the distillation process. Oil from a cheaper South American variety may be imported and blended, then sold as European.

Contraindications: None known.

PINE   Latin name: *Pinus sylvestris*

Family species: *Pinaceae*

Purchasing guide: **Color:** Pale yellow; **Viscosity:** Watery; **Aroma:** Crisp, clean, fresh, resinous

Countries of origin: USA, Scotland, Russia, France

Description: A tree, reaching 130 feet, with evergreen needles on branches extending from a straight trunk, with male and female cones.

Part used: Needles, twigs, and buds

Extraction method: Steam distillation

Yield: 0.1–0.5%

Most valuable uses: Rheumatism, muscular pain, muscular fatigue, bronchial infections, colds, coughs, general debility, mental exhaustion, asthma, sinus infections, cellulite, urinary problems

Therapeutic properties: Anti-infectious, anti-fungal, antiseptic, tonic, pectoral, expectorant, diuretic, balsamic, stimulant, depurative, restorative

Main chemical components: Sylvestrene, pinene, bornyl acetate, pumilone, dipentene, cadinene

Blends well with: Clary sage, cypress, lavender, rosemary, tea tree, juniper, lemon, grapefruit, eucalyptus (all), frankincense, marjoram, peppermint, ravensara, thyme linalol, bergamot, cedarwood, sandalwood

Interesting facts: Also known as "Scottish pine." Grows wild in all parts of Europe and Russia, and is extensively cultivated for wood, cellulose, tar, pitch, turpentine, and essential oil. The oil is used in medicines, food, confectionery, drinks, and men's toiletries. The tree is the source of edible pine kernels, which come from the cones. According to an ancient Egyptian cookbook, pine kernels were appreciated for their nutritional value.

Contraindications: Possible irritant to sensitive skins.

RAVENSARA   Latin name: *Ravensara aromatica*

Family species: *Lauraceae*

Purchasing guide: **Color:** Clear; **Viscosity:** Watery; **Aroma:** Slightly spicy, camphory, woody herbaceous

Country of origin: Madagascar

Description: Tree with strongly aromatic bark and dark, smooth evergreen leaves. It produces flowers and seeds, which are used as a spice.

Part used: Leaves and branches

Extraction method: Steam distillation

Yield: 1.0–1.5%

Most valuable uses: Colds, flu, bronchitis, diarrhea, fever, cold sores, chicken pox, measles, muscular pain, muscular fatigue, general tonic

Therapeutic properties: Antiseptic, anti-viral, anti-toxic, antibiotic, anti-infectious, expectorant, febrifuge

Main chemical components: 1,8-Cineole, a-pinene, b-pinene, p-caryophyllene, terpenyle acetate, b-caryophyllene

Blends well with: Bay, benzoin, bergamot, black pepper, cardamom, cedarwood, clary sage, cypress, eucalyptus (all), geranium, frankincense, ginger, grapefruit, lavender, mandarin, marjoram, lemon, palmarosa, pine, rosemary, sandalwood, tea tree, thyme linalol, thyme red

Interesting facts: The bark of the tree is used to make a local rum. The seeds are known as Madagascan nutmeg and are used in cooking and medicines.

Contraindications: None known.

ROSE MAROC (Rose de Mai)   Latin name: *Rosa centifolia*

Family species: *Rosaceae*

Purchasing guide: **Color:** Deep reddish-orange; **Viscosity:** Medium; **Aroma:** Deep, soft, hypnotic, honey-spicy rose. *Often adulterated during extraction with other rose species, or palmarosa or geranium.*

Countries of origin: Morroco, Algeria, Tunisia, France, Egypt

Description: Rose bush growing to six feet high. In Morocco the bush is trained to grow vertically because it produces hundreds of blossoms in this way.

Part used: Fresh flower heads

Extraction method: Enfleurage and solvent extraction

Yield: 0.12%

Most valuable uses: Infertility, female reproductive problems, depression, anxiety, headaches, nervous tension, circulation, skin care, emotional crisis, scarring, general tonic

Therapeutic properties: Anti-infectious, antiseptic, astringent, tonic, stimulant, aphrodisiac, emollient, nervine, cytophylactic

Main chemical components: Phenyl-ethanol, Citronellol, Geraniol, Nerol, Stearopten, Farnesol

Blends well with: Jasmine, neroli, geranium, sandalwood, clove, palmarosa, lemon, ginger, ylang ylang, mandarin, patchouli, frankincense, cardamom, coriander, bay, benzoin

Interesting facts: This oil is not produced by steam distillation because the yield in this manner from *rosa centifolia* is too slight. There are 5,000 varieties of rose, only a few of which have a distinct fragrance. The species here is known as the "light pink cabbage rose;" the name *centifolia* indicating the large number of petals. The species was introduced into Morocco by the Arabs in the 7th century. Now most rose production takes place south of the Atlas Mountains, adjacent to the desert, between 3,000–5,000 feet above sea level. Traditionally, the rose bush was grown as a dense hedge around wheat and bean fields and domestic gardens, and between rows of trees. Nowadays, in addition, roses are grown on a commercial basis in huge fields.

Contraindications: None known.

ROSE OTTO   Latin name: *Rosa damascena*

Family species: *Rosaceae*

Purchasing guide: Color: Clear with slight green-ish tint; **Viscosity:** From watery to crystalline, when warm or cold respectively; **Aroma:** Flowery, rosy, lemony, fresh. *The different species provide variety in aroma, between* R damascene *(Damask rose),* R Centifolia *(Cabbage rose), and* R Indica *(Tea Rose), and between hybrids.*

Countries of origin: Bulgaria, Turkey, India, France

Description: Bush growing to four feet, flowering once a year. The flowers are pink, sometimes white, but the white are not used in essential oil production. (The leaves also contain a quite different essential oil, although it is not as common as the flower head oil).

Part used: Fresh flowers, picked before 8 A.M.

Extraction method: Steam distillation. *The aroma can be damaged if the heat at distillation is too high.*

Yield: 0.02–0.05%

Most valuable uses: Female reproductive problems, infertility, scarring, poor circulation, childbirth, aphrodisiac, nervous tension, calming, emotional crisis, general tonic, skin problems, skin care.

Therapeutic properties: Anti-infectious, tonic, astringent, aphrodisiac, cicatrisive, cytophylactic, pectoral, antidepressant, sedative, calmative, haemostatic, emollient, antiseptic

Main chemical components: Citronellol, Geraniol, Nonadecan, Nerol, Nonadecen, phenyl-ethanol, Farnesol

Blends well with: Jasmine, neroli, geranium, lavender, clary sage, sandalwood, lemon, chamomile roman, mandarin, ylang ylang, petitgrain, vetiver, bergamot, patchouli, benzoin

Interesting facts: *Rosa* comes from the Greek *roden,* meaning "red," as the ancient rose was thought to have been crimson. In myth, the rose was supposed to have sprung from the blood of Adonis (some accounts say Venus). Although the oil is obliquely referred to in the ancient Indian Ayurvedas and is mentioned by Homer in the *Iliad,* the first known rose oil distilleries existed in the year 1612 in Shiraz, part of Persia. The rose produces rose oil, rose attar/otto and rose water. It takes about 10,000 lbs. of flowers to make one lb. of rose oil.

Contraindications: None known.

ROSEMARY   Latin name: *Rosmarinus officinalis*

Family species: *Labiatae (Labiaceae)*

Purchasing guide: Color: Clear; **Viscosity:** Watery;
Aroma: Camphor-like, woody, herbaceous, powerful.
*The rosemary oil from Corsica is softer, having less
camphor and more esters. Moroccan rosemary is more
fresh-smelling, due to the cineole.*

Countries of Origin: France, Spain, Morocco, Tunisia

Description: Bush growing to four feet, with twisted stems
and long, thin branches growing spike-like leaves and blue
flowers.

Part used: Leaves and twigs

Extraction method: Steam distillation of flowering tops, for no
more than two hours

Yield: 1.0–2.0%

Most valuable uses: Muscular pain, rheumatism, arthritis,
muscular weakness, constipation, coughs, colds, bronchitis,
helps eliminate toxins, memory enhancement, overwork,
general debility, infections, overindulgence, hangovers, acne,
exhaustion, poor circulation, cellulite, skin care, hair care,
migraine, headaches, sinus problems, general tonic

Therapeutic properties: Antiseptic, anti-spasmodic, stimulant,
analgesic, rubefacient, antidepressant, anti-toxic, pectoral,
vulnerary, carminative, emmenagogue, diuretic, stomachic,
antitussive, decongestant

Main chemical components: 1,8-Cineole, beta Pinene,
Camphor, Camphene, Borneol, Bornyl acetate

Blends well with: Lemon, geranium, lavender, peppermint,
tea tree, thyme linalol, grapefruit, clary sage, palmarosa,
juniper, cypress, pine needle, bergamot, black pepper, cedarwood, eucalyptus (all), frankincense, mandarin, marjoram,
ravensara, oregano, naiouli, litsea cubeba, basil

Interesting facts: Considered sacred by ancient Egyptians,
Hebrews, Greeks, and Romans. All ancient healers used rose-
mary, including the Swiss 16th century doctor and alchemist,
Paracelsus. Many mentioned its ability to heighten memory.
The flowers are a source of an excellent honey. Used extensively
in hair lotions and for the prevention of premature balding.

Contraindications: Not to be used in pregnancy. Not to be
used by people with epilepsy.

SANDALWOOD   Latin name: *Santalum album*

Family species: *Santalaceae*

Purchasing guide: Color: Pale yellow to pale gold; **Viscosity:** Viscous; **Aroma:** Warm balsamic rich woody. *Other species produce an oil which is similar in smell only (not in terms of therapeutic values) — the African* Osyris tenuifolia *plant, the Australian* Antalum spicatum, *and the West Indian* Amyris balsamifera.

Countries of origin: India (Mysore province), Indonesia, New Caledonia

Description: An evergreen tree with bunches of reddish-yellow flowers growing at altitudes of 2,000–3,000 feet. The tree can grow up to 65 feet high and is hemiparasite, sucking its nourishment from other trees roots. It can take thirty to fifty years for the tree to reach full maturity, when it is cut and distilled.

Part used: Heartwood and root

Extraction method: Steam distillation of chipped wood

Yield: 4–6.5%

Most valuable uses: Bronchitis, catarrh, coughs, fluid retention, bladder infections, throat infections, depression, cystitis, scarring, anxiety, nervous tension, acne, skin care, aphrodisiac, relaxing, stress, tension, chest infections, nausea, nervous exhaustion, chronic illness

Therapeutic properties: Antiseptic, antidepressant, diuretic, tonic, aphrodisiac, astringent, emollient, calmative, anti-infectious, decongestant

Main chemical components: Sesquiterpinol Santalol, Santenonol, Teresantalal, Borneol, Santalene

Blends well with: Black pepper, geranium, grapefruit, frankincense, fennel, myrrh, benzoin, patchouli, petitgrain, orange, clary sage, palmarosa, ylang ylang, mandarin, lavender, lemon, clove, chamomile roman, rose maroc, rose otto, neroli, jasmine, vetiver

Interesting facts: The documented use of sandalwood goes back 4,000 years. The caravans of ancient Egypt, Greece, and Rome brought it back from Asia. Swahra yoga recommends it for the union of the senses; Tantric yoga recommends it to awaken sexual energy. Used in ancient China for sexual disease, and by Ayurvedic doctors for urinary disorders. It is used to make furniture and caskets because it is insect resistant.

Contraindications: None known.

SPIKENARD — Latin name: *Nardostachys jatamansi*

Family species: *Valerianaceae*

Purchasing guide: **Color:** Pale yellow; **Viscosity:** Medium; **Aroma:** Heavy, warm, peaty, musty

Countries of origin: India, Nepal, Bhutan, Japan

Description: A perennial herb on a straight stem, green leaves, and small, pinky-mauve bell-shaped flowers.

Part used: Root

Extraction method: Steam distillation

Yield: 1–3%

Most valuable uses: Insomnia, physical tension, stress-related conditions, anxiety, nervous tension, hysteria, general aches, menstrual problems, backache

Therapeutic properties: Antiseptic, antibiotic, anti-fungal, anti-inflammatory, calmative, sedative, anti-infectious

Main chemical components: Valeranone, Jonon, Tetramethyloxatricylodecanol, Methylthymyl-ether, Cineol-1,8

Blends well with: Lavender, pine, clove, lemon, clary sage, palmarosa, juniper, cypress, geranium, rose maroc, neroli, frankincense, myrrh, patchouli, vetiver

Interesting facts: Related to valerian. Known in ancient times as "nard." In Chapter 12 of the *Book of John* in the Bible it says, "Then took Mary a pound of ointment of spikenard, very costly, and anointed the feet of Jesus." Wealthy Roman women used it in beauty preparations. Used in India to encourage hair growth, and darken the color.

Contraindications: None known.

TAGETES   Latin name: *Tagetes glandulifera, T minuta*

Family species: *Asteraceae (Compositea)*

Purchasing guide: Color: Yellowish to reddish-amber; **Viscosity:** Medium, but turning thick and even gel-like if exposed to the air; **Aroma:** Slightly bitter, fruity, herbaceous

Countries of origin: Argentina, South Africa, France, Nepal, India

Description: A weed which can grow up to six feet in the wild, with deep-green, divided leaves and numerous yellowish-orange flowers which look like daisy heads.

Part used: Leaves, stalks and flowers, picked when the seeds are just starting to form

Extraction method: Steam distillation

Yield: 0.1–0.5%

Most valuable uses: Athlete's foot, corns, calluses, bunions, catarrh, coughs, chest infections, parasitic infestations, fungal infestations

Therapeutic properties: Anti-infectious, anti-fungal, antibiotic, anti-spasmodic, emmenagogue, mucolytic, anti-parasitic, antiseptic

Main chemical components: Ocimenes, Dihydro Tageton, Dihydotagetone, Thymol

Blends well with: Bergamot, clary sage, lemon, lavender

Interesting facts: The leaves and flowers are a good insect repellent. The smell is similar to the African marigold. It is hung in doorways as a fly and mosquito deterrent in Africa, and as mattress stuffing to keep out bugs and pests. In Uganda it is used to treat and deter disease and insects. The oil in a 5% dilution has been used to kill maggots in open wounds as well as other ticks and parasites. Tagetes is an ingredient of many foot treatment preparations. The species *Tagetes Lucida* from Mexico is used as an hallucinogenic by traditional shamans.

Contraindications: Not to be used in pregnancy. Not to be used on children under 16 years. May cause skin irritation on sensitive skins. May cause photosensitivity.

TEA TREE Latin name: *Melaleuca alternifolia*

Family species: *Myrtaceae*

Purchasing guide: Color: Very pale yellow; **Viscosity:** Watery; **Aroma:** Sharp. spicy, warm, camphorous. *Because demand outstrips supply, tea tree oil is sometimes adulterated with other species of Melaleuca, of which there are many varieties. This is allowed by the authorities but no data exists to verify the efficacy of these blended oils.*

Country of origin: Australia

Description: Tree, cut back to bush size, about four feet on average. The leaves are slender and about three inches long.

Part used: Leaves and twigs

Extraction method: Steam distillation

Yield: 1.8%

Most valuable uses: Rashes, insect bites, nail fungus, dermatitis, ringworm, thrush, head lice, sore throats, boils, bronchial congestion, scabies, ulcers, wounds, arthritis, cold sores, acne, fatigue, useful for all infections

Therapeutic properties: Anti-infectious, antibiotic, balsamic, anti-fungal, anti-viral, anti-parasitic, vulnerary, anti-inflammatory, expectorant, immunostimulant, decongestant, analgesic, antiseptic

Main chemical components: Terpinene-4-ol, Paracymene, Caryophyllene, Gamma-Terpinene, Alpha-terpinene

Blends well with: Basil, bergamot, black pepper, lavender, rosemary, lemon, chamomile roman, chamomile german, eucalyptus globulus, eucalyptus radiata, clary sage, juniper, cypress, pine, marjoram, oregano, peppermint, ravensara, thyme linalol, thyme red

Interesting facts: Aboriginal Australians used this plant for many medicinal purposes. In World War II cutters and producers of tea tree were exempt from military service until enough essential oil had been accumulated. It was issued to each soldier and sailor for them to treat tropical infections and other problems of warfare, including wounds.

Contraindications: None known.

THYME
(red and chemotype linalol)
Latin name: *Thymus vulgaris*

Family species: *Labiatae*

Purchasing guide: Color: Red thyme is light reddish-brown to amber; Thyme linalol is pale yellow; **Viscosity (both):** Medium to watery; **Aroma:** Red thyme is sharp, woody herbaceous. Thyme linalol has a softer, woody herbaceous aroma. *The species known as thyme linalol is gentler and therefore can be used on children.*

Countries of origin: France, Spain

Description: Perennial dwarf shrub growing to only 12 inches high, with woody stems, tiny slightly woolly leaves, and pink-to-lilac flowers.

Part used: Flowering tops

Extraction method: Steam distillation

Yield: 0.7–1.0%

Most valuable uses: All infections including viral infections, mucous congestion, colds, flu, muscular pains, arthritis, obesity, bronchitis, coughs, general debility, poor circulation, gout, physical exhaustion, throat infections, muscular debility, anorexia, acne, gum infections, thrush, verrucas, warts

Therapeutic properties: Antibiotic, pectoral, analgesic, expectorant, antiseptic, balsamic, anti-infectious, anti-viral, stimulant, tonic, rubefacient, diuretic, emmenagogue, vermifuge, anti-venomous, anti-putrescent, anti-spasmodic, anti-fungal, immunostimulant

Main chemical components: 6-isopropyl-m-cresol, Terpenoid phenol thymol, isomer carvacrol, cymol, linalool, camphene

Blends well with: Geranium, grapefruit, clary sage, palmarosa, lemon, rosemary, eucalyptus (all), cypress, pine, tea tree

Interesting facts: Thyme was used medicinally by the Egyptians, Greeks, and Romans. Most present-day research has centered on thyme's ability as an antibacterial and anti-infectious agent, even when diffused in the air. There are several species of thyme oil in use, and although the strongest is red thyme and the gentlest is linalol, their uses are the same. The difference is not in what they both do, but in their relative strength.

Contraindications: Neither thymes are to be used in pregnancy. Not to be used in baths. Red thyme not to be used on children. Red thyme can be a mucus membrane and skin irritant so never use neat on the skin. Red thyme is one the best anti-infectious agents when diffused in the atmosphere.

VETIVER	Latin name: *Vetiveria zizanoides*

Family species: *Gramineae (Graminaceae)*

Purchasing guide: **Color:** Amber to olive; **Viscosity:** Viscous; **Aroma:** Earthy, musty. *Should have softness and body.*

Countries of origin: Java (Indonesia), Haiti, Reunion, India, Angola, Zaire, New Guinea, Brazil

Description: Perennial grass growing to six feet high with long, rhizomatous roots

Part used: Washed, dried, sliced, or ground roots

Extraction method: Steam distillation

Yield: 0.5%

Most valuable uses: Rheumatism, circulatory tonic, menstrual problems, stress, tension, calming, nervous tension, cleansing, overindulgence

Therapeutic properties: Antiseptic, tonic, stimulant, immunostimulant, emmenagogue, anti-spasmodic, sedative, anti-parasitic, nervine

Main chemical components: Benzoic acid, Furfural, Vetiverol, Vetivenol, Vetiveron, Sesquiterpene

Blends well with: Patchouli, sandalwood, orange, lemon, mandarin, grapefruit, eucalyptus citriodora, litsea cubeba, yuzu, melissa, geranium, ylang ylang, lavender, clary sage, jasmine, rose maroc, bergamot, black pepper, coriander, ginger, lemongrass

Interesting facts: The roots are interwoven with floor matting, window coverings, etc, giving rooms a fragrance and deterring insects. The oil is used in chypre and oriental type perfumes, and soaps, toiletries, etc. Growing the plant protects against soil erosion.

Contraindications: None known.

YLANG YLANG   Latin name: *Canangium odorata forma genuina*

Family species: *Anonaceae*

Purchasing guide: Color: Pale yellow; **Viscosity:** Medium to watery; **Aroma:** Sweet, intense, balsamic, floral. *An essential oil is also produced by* Cananga odorata forma macrophylla, *which gives the oil cananga. This has a harsher, leathery-burnt ylang ylang odor which is often sold in place of ylang ylang.*

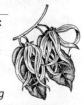

Countries of origin: Comoros Islands (Madagascar), Reunion, Haiti, Zanzibar

Description: A tree growing over 60 feet high, with large, drooping yellow flowers. At first these are green, covered with white hair and without fragrance, but after about 20 days the color changes to white, then yellow with a strong odor.

Part used: Fresh, fully developed flowers, best picked at dawn

Extraction method: Steam distillation. As the flowers can be distilled several times, there are several qualities of essential oil, the finest is known as "extra." When the flowers are distilled for the second time this produces grade "1," and so on to grade "3." Only "extra" has the qualities required for aromatherapy.

Yield: 1.5–2%

Most valuable uses: Nervousness, physical exhaustion, depression, stress, aphrodisiac, skin care, nervous tension, irritability, anxiety, PMS, regulates circulation, uterine tonic, hair growth

Therapeutic properties: Sedative, antiseptic, aphrodisiac, nervine, antidepressant, calmative, anti-seborrheic

Main chemical components: Linalol, Geranyl acetate, Benzyl benzoate, B-caryophyllene, Benzyl Acetate

Blends well with: Lemon, mandarin, palmarosa, yuzu, litsea cubeba, eucalyptus citriodora, clove, orange, ginger, sandalwood, jasmine, neroli, bergamot, chamomile roman, clary sage, patchouli, jasmine, rose maroc, rose otto, petitgrain, vetiver, grapefruit

Interesting facts: Ylang means "flower of flowers," sometimes called "the perfume tree." The flowers are picked early in the morning. They are also laid in between cloth to impart their fragrance. Used in coconut oil, ylang ylang is called macassar oil and used in hair preparations. The oil is used in confectionery, as well as in perfumery.

Contraindications: None known.

YUZU — Latin name: *Citrus junos*

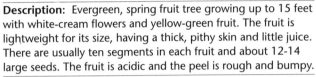

Family species: *Rutaceae*

Purchasing guide: **Color:** Yellowy-orange; **Viscosity:** Watery; **Aroma:** Unique blend of fresh tangerine/lime/ grapefruit/lemon

Country of origin: Japan

Description: Evergreen, spring fruit tree growing up to 15 feet with white-cream flowers and yellow-green fruit. The fruit is lightweight for its size, having a thick, pithy skin and little juice. There are usually ten segments in each fruit and about 12-14 large seeds. The fruit is acidic and the peel is rough and bumpy.

Part used: Peel of the fruit

Extraction method: Cold-pressed

Yield: 0.7–0.8%

Most valuable uses: General tonic, antiseptic, nervous tension, stress, anxiety, cystitis, constipation, cleansing, nervous stomach cramps, neuralgia, post-viral problems, convalescence.

Therapeutic properties: Tonic, stimulant, antibiotic, anti-infectious, anti-putrescent, diuretic, anti-viral, calmative, nervine, sedative, antiseptic, analgesic, anti-fungal

Main chemical components: Limonene, y-terpinene, B-Phellandrene, Myrcene, Linalol, a-pinene, Terpinolene

Blends well with: Basil, bay, benzoin, bergamot, black pepper, cardamom, cedarwood, chamomile roman, clary sage, clove, coriander, cypress, eucalyptus citriodora, ginger, jasmine, lavender, marjoram, orange, lemon, patchouli, palmarosa, petitgrain, pine, ravensara, rose maroc, rosemary, sandalwood, vetiver, ylang ylang

Interesting facts: First recorded in China in 237 B.C, by Pu-Wei in his book *Spring and Summer Annals.* Although the tree is still cultivated sparingly in North-Central China, it is now more extensively grown in Japan, where it was introduced over 1,000 years ago. Yuzu is very cold-hardy and is therefore grown in areas too cold for other citrus fruits. It is very resistant to rot. Yuzu is grown for its fruit and also as a rootstop for other citrus varieties. In Japan the rind, juice, and fruit are used extensively as flavorings — especially in vinegars, soups, seafood dishes, sauces, pickles, and salads. It is also used in religious ceremonies by Shinto priests for purification before prayer. Make into a soft drink popular in South America.

Contraindications: None known.

$\mathscr{A}$ppendix

SUPPLIERS

Essentially Yours Ltd, 371 "A" London Road, Westcliff On Sea, Essex SS07HT, England Telephone: 01702 390625, Fax: 01702 391344 *Essentially Yours Ltd* provides a comprehensive mail order service to the U.S., supplying essential oils and products, diffusers, etc., to both professionals and the public.

NORTH AMERICAN SUPPLIERS

Essentially Yours Canada
Deborah Arnie
Anahata Center, 6240 Constable Drive, Richmond, British Columbia V7E 3Y2, Canada
Telephone: (604) 241-9774 Fax: same as telephone Voicemail (604) 473 6097

Casandra Hawkins
934 Arkell Street, Ottawa, Ontario K2B 5R3, Canada, Telephone (613) 829 2684

Cyre Muellar
22 Farnham Drive, Calgary, Alberta T2H 1C6, Canada, Telephone: (403) 255 8266

Aroma Vera Inc
P.O. Box 3609, Culver City, California 90231
Telephone (800) 669 9514

Original Swiss Aromatics
Pacific Institute of Aromatherapy, PO Box 606, San Rafael,
California 94915, Telephone: (415) 459 3998

Singapore Supplier
Bodi-Mind Lifestyle PTE Ltd
8 Lowrong Bakar Bato, #03-01 Kolam Ayer Industrial Park,
Singapore 1334, Telephone: 748 6177, Fax: 743 3065

Mother & Baby
Essential Well Being
P.O. Box 160
Wokingham Berkshire RG11 3YX
England, Telephone: 01 734 791 737

Training

International Academy of Holistic Studies
P.O. Box 210, Romford, Essex, England RM7 7DW
Aromatherapy correspondence courses (international)

Aromatherapy Seminars
3389 So. Robinson's Place, Los Angeles, California 90034

Aromatherapy Organizations

International Federation of Aromatherapists
Stamford House, 2-4 Chiswick High Road, London W4
0TZ, England Telephone 0181 742 2605

National Association for Holistic Aromatherapy
P.O. Box 17622, Boulder, Colorado 80308-7622

The American Alliance of Aromatherapy
P.O. Box 750428, Petaluma, California 94975

**The American Phyto-Therapy and Aromatherapy
Association**
P.O. Box 3679, South Pasadena, California 91031

The International Federation of Aromatherapists
(Australia)
1/390 Burwood Road, Hawthorn, Victoria 3122, Australia,
Telephone: (613) 819 2502, Fax: (613) 819 2399

SELECTED BIBLIOGRAPHY

Balz, Rodolphe, *Les Huiles Essentielles*, Crest: R Balz, 1986

Bardeau, Fabrice, *La Medecine par les Fleurs*, Paris: Editions Robert Laffont, 1976

Bernadet, Marcel, *La Phyto-aromatherapie Pratique*, St Jean de Braye: Editions Dangles, 1983

Duraffourd, *The Best of Health, Thanks to Essential Oils*, Perigny: La Vie Claire, 1984

Franchomme, P., Pénoél, D., *L'aromathérapie Exactement*, Limoges: Roger Jollois Editeur, 1990

Gattefossé, René, *Gattefossé's Aromatherapy*, Safron Walden: C. W. Daniel Co., 1993

Grieves, Maud, *A Modern Herbal*, London: Jonathan Cape, 1979

Guenther, Ernest, *The Essential Oils* (6 volumes), Malabar, FL: Robert E. Krieger, 1952 (Reprint 1975)

Lautié, Raymond, and Passebecq, Andre, (trans. Dudley) *Aromatherapy*, Wellingborough: Thorsons, 1979

Lavabre, Marcel F., *Aromatherapy Workbook*, Rochester: Healing Arts Press, 1990

Linskens H. F., and Jackson, J. F., *Essential Oils and Waxes*, New York: Springer Verlag, 1991

Poucher, W. A., *Perfumes, Cosmetics and Soaps* (3 volumes), London: Chapman and Hall, 1974

Scholes, Michael, *Aromatherapy: Answers to the Most Commonly Asked Questions*, Los Angeles: AromaPress International, 1993

Svendsen, A. Baerheim, and Scheffer, J. J. C., *Essential Oils and Aromatic Plants*, Boston: Martinus Nijhoff/Dr. W.

Junk, 1985

Tisserand, Robert, *Aromatherapy to Heal and Tend the Body*, Wilmot, WI: Lotus Light, 1989

Valnet, Jean, *The Practice of Aromatherapy*, Safron Walden: C.`   W. Daniel Co., 1986

Valnet, J., Duraffourd C., and Lapraz, J. C., *Phytotherapie & Aromathérapie*, Paris: Presses de la Renaissance, 1978

Worwood, Valerie Ann, *The Complete Book of Essential Oils and Aromatherapy*, San Rafael, CA: New World Library, 1991

Worwood, Valerie Ann, *Aromantics*, New York: Bantam Books, 1994

Worwood, Valerie Ann, *The Fragrant Mind*, London: Doubleday, 1995

Index

A

About the Author

Susan Worwood, MIFA Reg., is a professional aromatherapist trained in clinical aromatherapy by her sister Valerie Ann Worwood. She has worked extensively with Valerie in research projects and in her London clinic. Susan continues to practice aromatherapy while also running an essential oil company. She is an active member of the International Federation of Aromatherapists and The Aromatherapy Trades Council.

If you would like a catalog of our fine
books and cassettes, contact:

New World Library
58 Paul Drive
San Rafael, CA 94903
(415) 472-2100 • Fax (415) 472-6131
Or call toll free: (800) 227-3900